Save Your Brain

Save Your Brain

Simple steps and proven strategies
to reduce your risk of cognitive
decline – before it's too late

DR GINNI MANSBERG

murdoch books
Sydney | London

Published in 2023 by Murdoch Books, an imprint of Allen & Unwin

Murdoch Books Australia
Cammeraygal Country
83 Alexander Street, Crows Nest NSW 2065
Phone: +61 (0)2 8425 0100
murdochbooks.com.au
info@murdochbooks.com.au

Murdoch Books UK
Ormond House, 26–27 Boswell Street, London WC1N 3JZ
Phone: +44 (0) 20 8785 5995
murdochbooks.co.uk
info@murdochbooks.co.uk

 A catalogue record for this book is available from the National Library of Australia

A catalogue record for this book is available from the British Library

ISBN 978 1 92261 634 0

Cover and text design by Mika Tabata
Typeset by Midland Typesetters
Printed and bound by CPI Group (UK) Ltd, Croydon, CR0 4YY

We acknowledge that we meet and work on the traditional lands of the Cammeraygal people of the Eora Nation and pay our respects to their elders past, present and future.

10 9 8 7 6 5

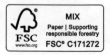

For Nana, Lonia (Leah) Liebhaber,
who gave unconditional love every day,
even when she hardly recognised us.
#nanagoals

Contents

Introduction

Back in February 2019, Australia's Royal Commission into Aged Care Quality and Safety started hearing over 10,000 submissions into what was happening to Australians living in care homes. It was shocking. Australians were horrified. How had we neglected our elderly so terribly? But after what seemed only a short period of time into the hearings, things got much worse for our elderly care home residents. COVID-19 started spreading through these facilities, not only killing some of the residents but forcing the elderly to isolate from loved ones and face their final weeks and months alone.

It was just so incredibly heartbreaking. While having all the empathy in the world, I admit that my first thought was: 'I never want to be in one of those places.'

But even before the royal commission and COVID-19 isolation, brain health was, and remains, a topic that weighs on the minds of many of us in midlife. A lot of us are now caring for parents or in-laws affected by dementia themselves. It's a stark reminder of our own brains' vulnerability.

Professor Ian Hickie is Co-Director, Health and Policy at the University of Sydney's Brain and Mind Centre. He is an internationally renowned researcher in clinical psychiatry and in brain health. He says people are right to start thinking about their brains in midlife. They're important! 'You know what you want to work in your 70s? Your brain. I don't mind if my knees don't work so much if I have my brain working!' he said. He says if you wear out your teeth, you can get false ones. 'Need new knees? We can do that for you! We also have amazing ways of renovating and repairing a worn-out heart. But your brain is precious. Once it's gone, it's gone for ever.'

For me this is personal. And with over 55 million people living with dementia around the world as of 2022, it may well be for you, too. My beloved nana spent her last few years in a nursing home with her brain deteriorating. Her (private, community-run) nursing home was nothing short of incredible, staffed with the most dedicated and loving humans on the planet. She was kept clean and retained her dignity until the day she died. She was also blessed because dementia didn't take her to a world of paranoia, fear or aggression. Five years after her cognition started to decline, she was alone when she took her last breath. The nurses rang my mum to tell her that Nana had slipped away quietly in her sleep. I wonder what that was like for her? Did she even know?

Ten years after losing my beautiful nana, Louis, my father-in-law, died of the same condition. Louis already had dementia when I met him. But things progressed rapidly and by the time he died, he was immobile and couldn't speak or feed himself. This was devastating for my husband, Daniel. He just adored and worshipped his dad and couldn't reconcile the dad in his heart with the man who left this world in his 80s.

Daniel has dementia on both sides of his family and we assume, without having done any gene tests, that dementia is going to touch him eventually. Like so many people I know, including many of my patients, friends and colleagues, we want desperately to hold back the tide and delay this as long as possible. Modelling done by Dr Ron Brookmeyer, the Dean of the UCLA Fielding School of Public Health, showed that delaying the onset of Alzheimer's disease by just five years across the board would reduce its prevalence in our community by 50 per cent. Five years! That's doable, right? But how do we do that? I've been determined to find out.

What is emerging from recent research is the relationship between your health in midlife and your risk of dementia. Dr Loren

Mowszowski is a clinical neuropsychologist who leads the Cognitive Training research stream within the specialised Healthy Brain Ageing Program at the Brain and Mind Centre, the University of Sydney. She says that the best time to turn your brain around is when you're in midlife: 40s, 50s and 60s. 'Later in life, in your 70s, the changes we can make in terms of lifestyle and co-morbidities are just slowing something down that's already started,' she says. 'But if we can target people in midlife, we have the best chance of being able to stop it before it starts or at least delay the onset of that decline.'

This is why I wrote this book. Because I wanted to work out exactly what Daniel, his siblings, my friends, my patients and I can do today to maximise our brain health and avoid dementia.

Now is the time to act to preserve your brain.

This book is jam-packed with pearls of wisdom, from small tweaks you can make, to the ways you can change your whole approach to life including diet, exercise, sleep and physical health. I delve into the studies and connect the dots between any given intervention and the proposed mechanisms behind it. I also present the opinions of a range of brain health experts from around the world. And perhaps most interestingly, I invite these experts to share what they do in their own lives to prevent cognitive decline. These men and women have spent an enormous amount of time and energy researching our brains and, in many cases, helping people suffering from dementia, so the decisions they make when it comes to their own brain health are revealing. You can see their comments throughout the book, or summarised on page 232.

Because the brain is complicated and neuroscience is so intricate, some sections of the book will be super dense. I hope they are not boring, but if you're tired you might want to skim through one or two of the chapters that are of less interest and skip to the end where I give you my takeaway tips.

All the strategies I suggest will make amazing differences to the structure of your body and mind. And, while warding off dementia, we'll throw in a lower risk of heart disease, diabetes, and even many cancers, for free! Every little change you make will help act as a prevention for all of these.

But let's be honest. None of us will be able to make every single change recommended in this book. Midlife is possibly *the* busiest time of your life. You are statistically likely to be in full-time work. You're likely to be juggling teenagers and/or ageing parents. The fifth decade is peak time for divorce in Australia. And our health is often taking a bit of a turn for the worse around this time, with many of us finding out we have high blood pressure, high cholesterol or even diabetes. If you're a woman, you might be in the middle of horrible peri and menopause symptoms, along with other common symptoms including mood swings and insomnia. You might have been told you need to do pelvic floor exercises three times a day to stop wetting your pants! And don't buy take-away! You need healthy home-cooked dinners from scratch. But how? When we're all just so busy?

You have to forgive yourself if you can't do every recommendation suggested in this book. Even if you make just three or four strategic changes that seem achievable, that's great. Don't beat yourself up for the changes you don't or can't yet make.

Ready? Let's do this!

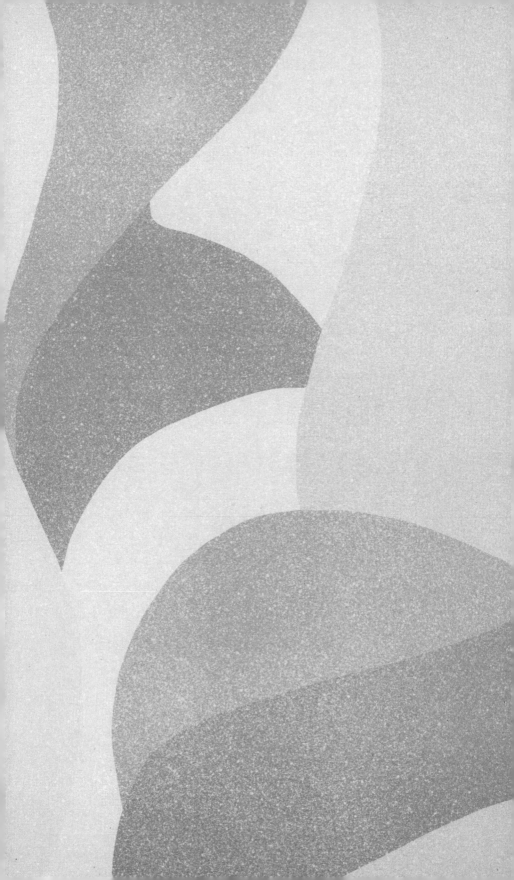

CHAPTER 1

Let me introduce your amazing brain

Before I launch into this chapter, I want to start with a caveat: the scientific concepts covered here are complex and can be really hard to get your head around, so feel free to skim through this section, or bypass it altogether, if science makes your eyes water. But it *is* a bit of a ready reckoner for some of the terms and explanations we'll discuss in the rest of the book. Rest assured, the rest of the book is nowhere near as hard!

Despite having done basic anatomy and physiology at uni, when I revisited this information again as a practising doctor there were things that I hadn't appreciated before. For example, just how *busy* the brain is. It accounts for 20 per cent of all of your body's oxygen consumption (more than any other organ), and sucks up 15 per cent of your heart's output, despite comprising only 2 per cent of the body's mass. I've also been amazed at how much we still don't know about it. Yes, with astounding advances in imaging techniques, our understanding of the brain and it's incredible functioning is growing all the time, but most of it remains shrouded in mystery.

I have been humbled and surprised by how *complex* the brain's workings are. Different parts of the brain intersect and communicate with each other in a dizzying number of ways. It takes multiple areas of the brain acting together to perceive things and respond. I think of the brain as a well-oiled organisation. While the different parts of the organisation might work on separate floors, that doesn't stop subgroups from forming and communicating effectively on certain projects.

On the following pages are some key terms and explanations that will be helpful when we are discussing brain function throughout this book.

1. **The brain is made up of two types of cells:** neurons and glial cells. Neurons send and receive nerve impulses or signals (see below for more details). Glial cells are the rest of the brain's cells. They're the brain's support cells, providing nutrition, maintenance, homeostasis, form myelin (a protective sheath around nerves) and facilitate signal transmission in the nervous system.

2. **There are three broad categories of glial cells.** Microglia, astrocytes and oligodendrocytes. Microglia are these amoeba-looking cells that travel around the brain searching for injuries and invaders. They're the primary actors in your brain's immune system, making up 10 per cent of your brains cells in number. Once a problem is detected, they zoom into the affected area to initiate a number of immune functions, producing an arsenal of cytotoxic and brain-cell-stimulating chemicals. They help clear dead or damaged brain cells and literally gobble up invading bugs. You can think of them as your brain's first responders when something goes wrong. The process of microglia activation acts as a kind of primer so that any subsequent insults results in an even greater microglia activation next time.

   Without microglia, your brain literally wouldn't function. But they are a bit of a double-edged sword. Microglia are great at recognising molecular patterns associated with microbes and cellular damage as bad and taking action to attack and then devour dead tissue. But the attack mode can be excessive and actually cause damage to healthy brain tissue, not just the unwanted bugs or toxins. This is important when we talk about what goes wrong with the brain in dementia in future chapters.

   Astrocytes are essential for maintaining the optimum chemical environment for neurons to work, including ensuring there are enough nutrients and oxygen.

   Oligodendrocytes are the cells that make the insulation system (the myelin that forms insulating and protective sheaths around the neurons), which ensures the neurons work properly.

Neurons are the chief workhorses of your brain, the cells that do all the thinking, moving, etc. A healthy adult brain has about 100 billion of them! More about them coming up.

3. **Grey matter.** This is made up of masses of cell bodies of neurons. Random fact: your grey matter volume actually peaks at about age six, before slowly declining. It is the grey area you see on the outside edges of a brain scan image.

4. **White matter.** This is made up of masses of axons of neurons. Here's another random fact: unlike your grey matter, your white matter grows more slowly, peaking at about age 30 before declining. It is the inside layer of white you see on brain scan images.

5. **Synapses.** The point where nerves meet and pass information to each other. This is done by tiny bursts of chemicals that are released by one neuron and detected by the others in that synapse. Your brain has about 100 trillion synapses in it!

6. **Neurotransmitters.** Your chemical messengers. They are molecules used by the nervous system to transmit messages between nerves or from nerves to muscles. They come in two flavours: excitatory (activate brain activity) and inhibitory (dampen it all down).

Your amazing neurons

Neurons use a combination of electrical impulses and chemicals to transmit information between each other, ultimately linking different parts of your brain to each other and to the rest of your body.

Neurons are long and tube-shaped so that nutrients and other essential substances can easily travel through the centre to different parts of the neuron. They have three basic parts: a cell body, an axon and a dendrite. Within the cell body is a nucleus containing all the genes, which is the cockpit driving each cell's activities. The axon looks like a long tail and transmits messages from the cell by sending the electrical and chemical messengers outbound. Dendrites look like the branches of a tree coming out of the cell body and they receive messages into the neuron. The tiny space where dendrites meet axons of adjacent neurons is called the synapse. This process is very energy intensive requiring *lots* of glucose.

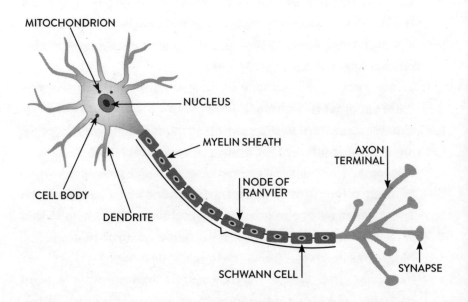

The function and survival of neurons depend on several key biological processes:

- **Communication.** Each chemical 'neurotransmitter' released from an axon into the synapse binds to a specific receptor site on the adjacent dendrite. This process triggers chemical or electrical signals that either stimulate or inhibit the activity of the neurons receiving the signal. One neuron may have up to 7000 connections with other neurons. Anything that interferes with the neurons being able to communicate with each other can harm the neurons.
- **Metabolism.** Generating and receiving signals is hungry work requiring huge amounts of oxygen and glucose, which are provided by blood vessels. No wonder the brain uses a whopping 20 per cent of all the energy used by the human body. Lose that constant supply of energy and your neurons run into problems.

- **Repair.** In contrast with the cells in the rest of your body, neurons can live more than 100 years each. Instead of dying off and being replaced, the cells around them are constantly modifying, pruning and repairing. That includes pruning back or growing extra connections between specific neurons and developing new synapses. This process is how we learn and code memories, as well as repair unwell neurons.

The brain's anatomy

Let's launch into your brain's anatomy, which is the structure of the brain that you would see if looking at a scan or 3D model. Random fact: a male brain weighs about 1336 grams, while a female brain comes in at about 1198 grams, but this difference in weight has absolutely no effect on function or intelligence.

The brain can be divided into three separate parts: the forebrain (front), the midbrain (middle) and the hindbrain (back).

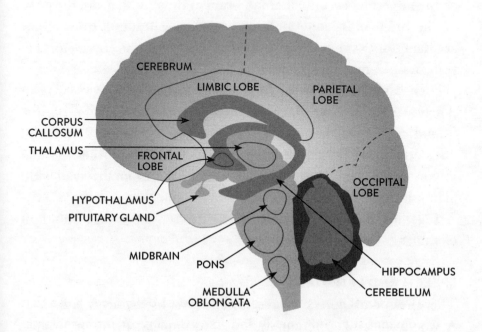

The forebrain

The forebrain is the largest and most highly developed part of the human brain. It is divided into two hemispheres, left and right, and they're connected by a bundle of neurons, which is called the corpus callosum.

The forebrain's main structure is the cerebrum which directs all the conscious motor functions of the body, like walking or picking up an apple. The outer layer of the cerebrum is called the cortex (consisting of grey matter) and the inner layer (white matter). There are four lobes in each cortex, the frontal lobe, parietal lobe, temporal lobe, occipital lobe (so eight lobes altogether).

It's worth looking at each of these. Mainly because when we discuss different studies and they refer to different parts of the brain that shrink, grow or get damaged, you'll know what we are referring to.

FRONTAL LOBES (AKA THE FRONTAL CORTEX)

The frontal lobes sit at the front of the cerebrum. They happen to be the largest lobes in the human brain and, sadly, they are the part of the brain most commonly injured during trauma, from a car accident, for example. They can be thought of as the conductors of your brain's amazing orchestra.

Each frontal lobe has multiple distinct areas in it, each with a different role to play. The prefrontal cortex is the section of the frontal cortex that lies at the very front of the brain. Tucked in just behind that is the premotor cortex. And behind that sits the motor cortex, which is the primary area of our brain involved with planning and executing voluntary movements.

Together, the different parts of the frontal lobes do a number of things.

SPEECH AND LANGUAGE

The prefrontal cortex is responsible for higher-level thinking. A whole stack of different studies have implicated the prefrontal cortex in your ability to speak, especially your narrative expression and your verbal fluency. The frontal lobe has an area called Broca's area that is essential for speaking. In a nutshell, Broca's area interprets the inputs from the temporal cortex going out to the motor cortex where the actual speaking happens.

PERSONALITY

The frontal lobes are also what cause you to be inhibited and not just act out at every impulse you have. They get shut off by alcohol and that's what leads to impulsive behaviour. We know there are marked personality changes that can happen after a frontal lobe injury. There was a famous case written about in the medical literature in 1848 when a man called Phineas Gage, who was apparently a gentle, polite, sociable young man was injured when a large iron rod was driven through his eye into his prefrontal cortex. After the injury, he became immediately insensitive, behaved socially inappropriately, and was altogether completely irrational.

Frontal lobe injuries classically cause:

- executive disturbances
- disturbed social behaviour
- emotional dysregulation
- being unemotional and having very low energy
- distress
- poor decision-making.

INTELLIGENCE

What makes somebody intelligent? It's a complicated topic. But studies based on functional MRI machines have found that the prefrontal cortex is involved with certain parts of brain function that determine intelligence, including verbal expression, memory, being able to tease out an abstract concept, and the ability to create and then execute a plan. The frontal cortex is also integral in anything to do with your ability to perceive spatial relationships between you and your environment, or to perform any task that needs visual information.

Damage to the frontal lobes (say from a stroke, a brain tumour or a car accident) can result in:

- loss of simple movement of specifically affected body parts
- loss of flexibility in thinking and becoming obsessed by a single idea (perseveration)
- loss of sequencing so that you can't work out how to do a task that requires a number of steps, such as preparing to go to work in the morning
- difficulty with problem solving
- inattention to the point of inability to focus on a task and to filter out distractions
- inability to express language
- mood fluctuations
- poor impulse regulation and changes in social behaviour
- reduced awareness and insight
- changes in personality.

MOVEMENT
People who have a stroke that affects their frontal lobe will be unable to move their arm or leg, or both, on the affected side. Interestingly if you have a stroke on the right half of your brain, the loss of function will be on the left, and vice versa.

MEMORY
The frontal lobes are critical to what we call prospective memory, which is a type of memory that involves remembering plans made, from a simple daily plan to future long-term plans.

Temporal lobes

Your temporal lobes are the second biggest part of the brain and sit behind the frontal lobes and below the parietal lobes. They're located on the sides of the brain at about ear level. Various parts of the temporal lobes are involved in everything from visual memory (which helps us recognise objects and faces), verbal memory (essential to understand language) and the ability to interpret other people's emotions and reactions.

The dominant temporal lobe, which for most of us is the left side, is involved in understanding language and learning and remembering verbal information.

The non-dominant lobe, which is typically the right temporal lobe, is involved in:

- learning and remembering non-verbal information (e.g. visuo-spatial material and music)
- sensorimotor planning
- creativity.

Damage to the temporal lobes can cause:

- difficulty in understanding words
- difficulty with identification and categorisation of objects
- difficulty in recognising faces
- difficulty learning and retaining new information
- problems with memory
- changes in interest in sexual behaviour
- emotional changes.

Parietal lobes

Your parietal lobes sit just behind your frontal lobes but above your temporal lobes and are connectors between various centres of the brain. Your parietal lobes are responsible for a huge and seemingly disparate range of things that we never think about that are really important. For example, they're involved in interpreting incoming sensory signals like touch, position, vibration, pressure, pain and temperature, along with coordination, body positioning in space, awareness of body differentiation (your right arm *feels* like your right arm!) and being able to distinguish right from left.

Damage to the parietal lobes can cause problems ranging from left–right confusion to being unable to recognise or monitor certain body parts depending on how much damage there is.

Occipital lobes

The occipital lobes are the smallest lobes in the cerebral cortex. They sit at the back of the brain, behind both the parietal and temporal lobes. These lobes are all about vision – specifically visual processing and interpretation using the signals coming in from the eyes.

Damage to the occipital lobes can result in finding it hard to identify the location or colour of an object, hallucinations, word blindness (which is the inability to recognise words) and difficulty in recognising the movement of an object, as well as struggles with reading and writing.

The limbic system

The limbic system is thought of as the primitive brain as it drives feelings as diverse as hunger, motivation, sex, mood, pain, pleasure and memory. Its purpose is essentially to process and make sense of the world. It consists of your hippocampus and amygdala in the temporal lobes, along with parts of the hypothalamus and thalamus. I think the limbic system is the *most* fascinating part of your brain. How can such a tiny and primitive part of the brain rule your emotions, happiness, loves and fears?

THE AMYGDALA

The amygdalae are a pair of small almond-shaped parts buried deep in the brain. They help control emotions and encode your memories, especially memories with high emotion. For example, if you have a really emotional experience, your amygdalae will tag that memory so you remember it more. I just want you to take a minute to think about that because it is just so profound. I know I remember events that once made me feel ashamed, guilty or really happy in detail. Thanks amygdala!

We know that in rats, and from a tiny study of people with epilepsy, if you stimulate the part of the amygdala involved in memory using a probe into the brain, it improves their memories. One day we might be able to do this for people without needing to stick a probe into the brain.

The amygdala is also the part of the brain that controls your 'fight or flight' response. Each amygdala receives inputs from all your senses, including visceral sensations (your guts, your breathing, etc), which combine to trigger a response.

Studies have shown that if you stimulate the amygdala, you get intense emotion, such as aggression, panic or fear.

THE HIPPOCAMPUS

The hippocampus, located in the temporal lobe, is where explicit or 'declarative memories' are formed and indexed for later access. Explicit memory is a type of long-term memory that involves remembering concepts, ideas and events that were learned or happened throughout life.

Recent research has shown that the hippocampus is not only critical for learning and memory but also for spatial navigation and emotional behaviour. It also helps regulate the hypothalamus (see page 14).

Like the amygdala, it has connections going to and from almost every other part of the brain. Unfortunately, it is very delicate. It is the earliest and most severely affected part of the brain in Alzheimer's disease and also in conditions like epilepsy.

THE HYPOTHALAMUS

The hypothalamus is a small region (about the size of an almond) buried deep within the brain that sits directly above the brainstem. It has two major functions: homeostasis and hormones. In terms of homeostasis, we are talking about things like regulating your body temperature and blood pressure, and keeping energy intake and expenditure at a fairly consistent level. The hypothalamus receives a steady stream of information from the body and acts a lot like the thermostat on a heater, dialling up and down various body functions to maintain a constant optimum level. It weaves its magic through control of the nerves called the autonomic nervous system and by the release of key hormones.

It controls your hormones through its regulation of the pituitary gland, also buried deep inside the brain. The hormones indirectly controlled by the hypothalamus include growth hormone (growth), follicle-stimulating hormone and luteinising hormone (involved in a woman's menstrual cycle), adrenocorticotropic hormone (stress/ fear response), thyroid-stimulating hormone and prolactin (milk production). In addition, your hypothalamus directly makes a couple of hormones. These include oxytocin and vasopressin or antidiuretic hormone (ADH). Oxytocin plays a role in childbirth and breast feeding, but research suggests it might also play a role in showing and feeling compassion and social bonding. ADH helps control urine output and regulate blood pressure (although it also seems to play a role in social and sexual behaviour).

THE THALAMUS

Sitting just above the midbrain and chiefly made up of grey matter, the thalamus acts as a relay station filtering information between the brain and body. It is made up of a bunch of different nuclei that are involved in relaying sensory signals to the appropriate part of the brain, as well as regulation of motor function and consciousness. It is also involved in mood and motivation.

The midbrain

The midbrain is the topmost portion of the brainstem. It is rich in nerves and their white matter tracts (or nerve highways), which are critical to motor control, as well as the auditory (hearing) and visual pathways, pain perception and more. Because it sits tucked in between the cerebral cortex, the cerebellum and the rest of the brainstem, it is a critical communication station that allows signals to be passed through and regulated.

There are three main parts of the midbrain: the colliculi (which process visual and auditory signals), the tegmentum (nuclei that communicate between the different parts of the brain and between brain and body) and the cerebral peduncles (transport signals from the cerebral cortex to the nerves around the body via the spinal column and are especially important for body coordination).

Sandwiched between these bundles and the tegmentum is a cluster of neurons called the substantia nigra, heavily pigmented cells that make the neurotransmitter dopamine. This critical little cluster of cells acts as a relay station for nerve signals that coordinate our movements. This is the area that is specifically damaged in Parkinson's disease.

The hindbrain

The hindbrain is made up of the upper part of the spinal cord, the brainstem, and a kind of ball that looks a bit like a brain coral as it is full of wrinkles, called the cerebellum. The hindbrain is vital as it controls all your body's essential functions like breathing and heart function.

Brainstem

Your brainstem is the most primitive part of your brain, but it is absolutely critical for life. It's not glamourous – it has nothing to do with personality, creativity, intellect or humour. However, it's the engine room of your body. The brainstem is the stalk that extends down from the brain to join up with the spinal cord. The spinal cord meets the brain through an opening in the skull called the foramen magnum. The lowest part of the brainstem is called the medulla oblongata, then further up lies the pons, and then the midbrain (see page 7).

Running throughout the brainstem is the reticular formation. This is a mesh-like system of nerves that helps your brain regulate your breathing, heart rate and blood pressure. Another mesh-like system running right through the brainstem is the spinothalamic tract, which helps the brain sense pain and temperature sensation, as well as crude touch.

MEDULLA OBLONGATA

The medulla contains the critical solitary nucleus, which is the first port in the brain to receive information about everything from taste and middle-ear sensations to blood flow, oxygen and carbon dioxide levels in the blood, from the heart and major blood vessels. It also receives signals from your gut. The thing that blows my mind is that this very same solitary nucleus that is busily receiving inputs from all over the body also sends signals out to communicate its finding to other parts of the brain. For example, it communicates with the limbic system that controls the emotional response to altered heart and respiratory rate numbers, and it plays a big bidirectional role in panic disorder. The solitary nucleus also sends signals out to the amygdala, contributing to memory. It communicates with the motor centres of the brain commanding it to cough, gag and vomit.

While we are on that topic, let me introduce the area postrema (aka the vomiting centre). It is designed to detect toxins in the blood or the brain itself and, unlike the rest of the brain, it is not protected by the so-called blood–brain barrier (see below) to keep out large molecules. That helps the area postrema detect toxins more easily. It also tells your body when to feel nausea and vomit.

PONS

The pons is named after the Latin word for 'bridge' because it connects the rest of the brainstem to the cerebral cortex. It sits above the medulla oblongata and underneath the midbrain, acting as a coordination centre for signals and communications that flow between the two brain hemispheres and the spinal cord.

THE CEREBELLUM

The cerebellum makes up only 10 per cent of the brain's volume, but it houses over 50 per cent of the total number of neurons in the brain. It basically coordinates and streamlines your movements. These might be initiated elsewhere in the brain, but this coordination is vital. If you see someone with cerebellar disease (alcohol abuse is the main culprit), they often struggle to walk properly and can't handle chopsticks or even point to things accurately. The cerebellum also plays a vital role in all the balance systems in your brain and, weirdly, it seems to play a role in language too, but not other cognitive functions.

Blood–brain barrier

There is an important barrier between the brain's blood vessels and the brain tissue. It turns out that the cells that line the brain's blood vessels are tightly packed together. The result is that only really small molecules, fat-soluble molecules, and some gases can pass freely into brain tissue. There are some larger molecules, such as glucose, that can enter the brain through piggy backing onto specialised transporter proteins (creatively called glucose transport protein or GLUT-1). The idea of the blood–brain barrier is to keep harmful toxins and bugs out but allow nutrients in. One side effect of the blood–brain barrier is keeping a lot of drugs *out* of the brain. It makes treating some brain diseases a real challenge.

I should point out that the brain has zero energy reserves and is completely dependent on a continuous and well-regulated delivery of oxygen and glucose through the cerebral blood supply.

If the blood supply to the brain goes down at any point, your brain doesn't have a lot of capacity to increase its own supply of vital nutrients.

Cerebrospinal fluid

Cerebrospinal fluid (CSF) is the roughly 150 ml of fluid that not only surrounds the brain and provides nourishment to your brain cells, but also plays a role in waste removal and protecting the brain. Your brain is constantly making then draining CSF at a rate of about 400 to 600 ml a day, completely turning over around five times a day. Here's another random fact: cerebrospinal fluid volume increases slowly from birth until about age 40 years, then increases rapidly after age 60 years, because that's when your brain is really shrinking, and the fluid moves in to fill the gaps.

The glymphatic system

I'd never heard of the glymphatic system until I started doing research for this book and spoke to Professor Sharon Naismith, who heads up the Healthy Brain Ageing Program at the Brain and Mind Centre at the University of Sydney. 'The glymphatic system controls CSF flow into the brain,' she told me. This system is a network of specialised vessels that clear toxins and other waste from the gaps between cells. And there are a *lot* of toxins there, mainly because your brain is just so metabolically active, it's spitting out a lot of waste all the time.

The glymphatic system also seems to help distribute glucose, lipids, amino acids and neurotransmitters through the brain. It has been referred to as the brain's 'front end' waste drainage system. How this system works and how it interconnects with the blood vessels, brain tissue and lymph vessels is only partly understood. But the glymphatic system seems to tip its waste into the CSF for ultimate disposal.

The glymphatic system operates mainly during sleep and is largely switched off when you're awake. Keep that in mind when we talk about the critical importance of sleep for brain health in Chapter 9.

Neurotransmitters of the brain

The brain's roughly 86 billion neurons communicate with each other by passing chemical messages at the synapse, which, as we have discussed, is the tiny gap between cells. Those chemical messages are molecules called neurotransmitters and although there are probably zillions of them, we've only identified around 60 of them. And just to keep us on our toes, neurons can synthesise and release more than one type of neurotransmitter over their lifetime.

There are two types of neurotransmitters. The first type is the small-molecule transmitters like dopamine and glutamate, which act directly on the neurons they're messaging. The second type is called neuropeptides, like insulin and oxytocin, which work more subtly, modulating or adjusting *how* cells communicate at the synapse.

ACETYLCHOLINE

This acts as a neurotransmitter through the body, stimulating muscle contractions and causing glands to secrete hormones. In the brain it acts more as a neuromodulator, helping other neurotransmitters do their thing.

GLUTAMATE

This important neurotransmitter is present in over 90 per cent of all brain synapses. It is critical for learning and memory as well as just normal brain functioning, and its level is tightly regulated. An excessive build-up of glutamate can damage neurons, and this has been linked to disorders including Parkinson's disease, stroke, seizures and increased sensitivity to pain.

GAMMA-AMINOBUTYRIC ACID (GABA)

GABA works to inhibit signalling between neurons. Drugs that increase GABA levels in the brain are used to calm the brain, for example to treat epileptic seizures, some tremors or as sleeping pills. Recently scientists have discovered that GABA helps with learning new information.

SEROTONIN

Serotonin is often called the 'calming chemical' as it brings on sleep. It is also involved in temperature regulation, appetite, memory and decision-making. Low levels of serotonin can cause sleep problems and depression, while too much serotonin can cause seizures.

DOPAMINE

Dopamine is often called the 'pleasure chemical' because it is released when you receive a reward sensation in response to something you have done or seen (like taste some chocolate!). Dopamine helps regulate mood and also helps regulate complex movements. It is involved in motivation, decision-making, movement, reward processing, attention, working memory and learning. Reduced amounts of dopamine in some parts of the brain leads to the rigid movements that characterise Parkinson's disease.

NORADRENALINE

This is both a hormone and a neurotransmitter. It has been linked to mood, vigilance, memory and stress.

So that's your brain. Phew! You made it! If you have more questions than answers, you're not alone. But I think this is all you need to plough through the next few chapters feeling more confident about what it all means. Especially when it comes to understanding and doing all you can to prevent unnecessary damage to your brain as you grow older.

Takeaways

- The brain is incredibly busy and uses 20 per cent of all the oxygen required by your body. This is more than any other organ in the body!
- The brain is made up of neuron cells (which transmit nerve messages) and glial cells (which remove waste products, provide nutrition and generate protective sheaths around nerves).
- There are three separate parts to the brain: the forebrain, the midbrain and the hindbrain. They contain all the neurons and pathways responsible for most of our most advanced functioning: speech, movement, language, personality, memory and emotional regulation.
- The brainstem sits below the lobes and extends into the spinal cord. It is responsible for all the unconscious bodily functions which keep us alive: breathing, heartbeat, blood pressure, sensation of touch and body temperature.

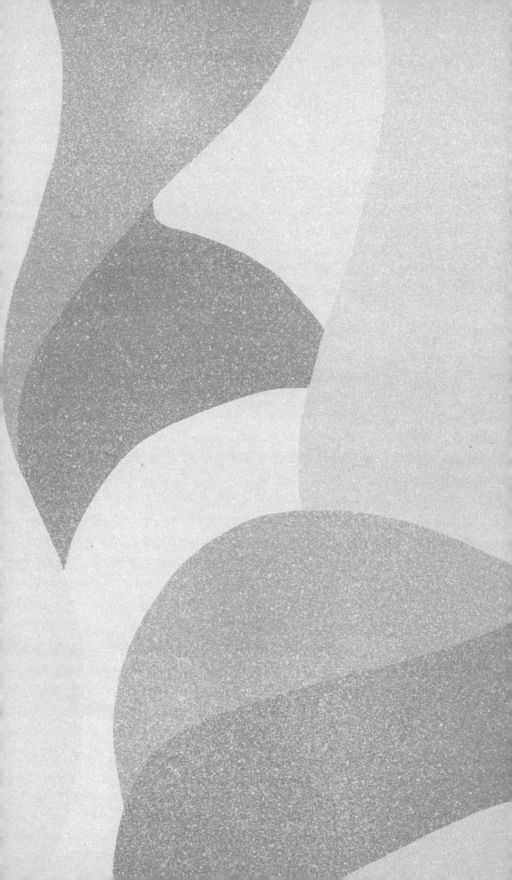

CHAPTER 2

The dementia lowdown

B ack in 2012, the Australian Government declared dementia the ninth identified national health priority area. That means that along with diabetes, mental health, cardiovascular disease, arthritis, obesity, asthma, cancer and injury prevention, and now COVID-19, it is one of the main areas of national health concern. **Today, we have made almost no inroads into reducing the impact of dementia.** It remains the number one cause of disability in Australians aged over 65 years and the second biggest cause of death overall. It is the number *one* cause of death in women over 65 in Australia and the UK, and number four in the US.

Dementia was traditionally seen as something that just happened as you got older, especially if you had the wrong genes. That was especially the case for the biggest cause of dementia, Alzheimer's disease. But there has been a sea change in thinking about the inevitability of dementia. Evidence is now mounting that 40–48 per cent of dementia risk is 'modifiable'.

While initially slow to take off, the idea that we can prevent or slow the progression of dementia is gaining momentum. Research in Australia shows that the 'modifiable' dementia risk factors include:

- physical inactivity (17.9 per cent)
- midlife obesity (17 per cent)
- low educational attainment in early life (14.7 per cent)
- midlife hypertension (13.7 per cent)
- depression (8 per cent)
- smoking (4.3 per cent)
- diabetes (2.4 per cent).

Other research adds to this list:

- hearing loss
- traumatic brain injury
- excessive alcohol use
- social isolation
- poor diet
- poor sleep
- air pollution.

It turns out that your lifestyle is probably a bigger contributor to dementia than your genes. But the biggest risk factor of all – getting older – isn't modifiable.

Your brain as you age

As you get older, your brain starts shrinking and it's the grey matter that shrinks most. (For more on grey matter see page 5.) White matter makes up the inside layer of your brain and is full of axons, which are responsible for connecting all the neurons between the different parts of the grey matter and then connecting the grey matter to different parts of the body. Since the neuronal cells in the grey matter are constantly working, they have a high oxygen demand. As a result, when the grey matter doesn't get enough oxygen, say because of an ageing blood supply, a problem with blood clotting (sometimes caused by inflammation) or any other cause, the cells will begin to die, leading to possible irreversible brain damage and loss of function. But this is quite different to dementia.

As you get older, you'll notice what we call cognitive slowing. One study found that a 20-year-old is 75 per cent faster than a 75-year-old at substituting symbols for numbers. While our vocabulary and general language skills remain pretty stable, the ability to find the right word might be a bit slower. Long-term memories are intact but we're not as good at forming new memories. Our working memory (responsible for things like remembering a set of instructions or a phone number) isn't as sharp as it used to be. You can still focus on a single task but multitasking seems a bit more difficult.

Our general knowledge and 'crystallised intelligence' (procedures and knowledge you have previously learned) are preserved but 'fluid intelligence' (the process of working out things that don't depend on things you have learned before) gets worse.

But that's not dementia. That's normal.

Is it dementia or just old age?

It's normal to forget where you left your keys. Start worrying if you're not quite sure what to do with your keys when you find them. It's normal not to be a natural finance guru. Start to worry when you don't pay your bills because you don't know how. Everyone forgets where they parked their car sometimes. Get worried if you can't remember how to exit the carpark at the local shopping centre.

So what actually is dementia?

Dementia is an umbrella term for symptoms caused by a loss of brain function that goes beyond what might be expected from the usual consequences of biological ageing. Symptoms include problems with memory, communicating, the ability to understand things like symbols and maps, problem solving and other comprehension issues. You can think of dementia as brain failure. The impairment in cognitive function is often packaged with (or preceded by) changes in mood, emotional regulation, behaviour or motivation. Most importantly, these problems make it hard to function in everyday life.

Dementia has many causes. And there are different types of dementia, with each one (initially) affecting different parts of the brain. But for all these differences they largely look the same in terms of symptoms.

Dividing up the different kinds of dementias into an arbitrary list, however, is problematic. According to Professor Ian Hickie, Co-Director of Health and Policy at the University of Sydney's Brain and Mind Centre, current research reveals that very few people with dementia have only one issue (or a traditional type of dementia) affecting their brains. If you check their brains under a microscope or through scans, there are usually multiple issues going on at once.

But here goes anyway.

Alzheimer's disease (AD)

Alzheimer's disease accounts for around two-thirds of all cases of dementia. Around 10 per cent of people have it by the time they hit 65 and this jumps to 32 per cent of 85-year-olds, although not every affected person realises they have it. It's important to say that we *still do not know* exactly what causes this brain disease.

What we do know is this: if you look at any brain affected by Alzheimer's disease, you'll see a build-up of toxic protein fragments called beta-amyloid (β-amyloid). This is a name you're going to read again and again in this book.

These β-amyloid fragments form plaques that sit outside the neuron cells. Not only do they eventually build up to a point where they damage the cells, they get stuck in the membranes between cells and in the synapse where neurons meet, which stops them from communicating with each other. β-amyloid plaques also build up in the blood vessels that supply the cells with blood, choking them off. The result is that brain cells are killed off.

β-amyloid is made when a protein called amyloid precursor protein (APP) is cut by two enzymes, called beta and gamma secretase. (Remember these because they're targets for drugs emerging now!) The cutting up of APP happens in a few different ways so that several different forms of β-amyloid are formed. The most toxic form, which is the major component in plaques, is called β-amyloid 42.

Dr Rachel Buckley is Assistant Professor of Neurology at Harvard University and Massachusetts General Hospital in the US. She tells me that β-amyloid builds up on the outside of the brain first. 'It will appear in the cortex, which is like the bark of the brain, and moves inward,' she explains. 'Although your brain can actually function pretty well when there's a lot of β-amyloid, once it hits a certain threshold it goes boom!'

In addition to the β-amyloid, you also see a build-up of twisted strands of another protein called tau (especially a form called phos-phorylated tau or p-tau) inside the neurons themselves. Tau itself isn't always toxic. In fact, it is an important chemical in its own right, as it helps stabilise the internal scaffolding of our neurons to keep an all-important tube shape. The shape allows nutrients to flow and messages to be passed from one cell to the next. But once the tau becomes phosphorylated, it changes the shape of the cell and stops it functioning like it should. In Alzheimer's disease, when this abnormal p-tau builds up, the tube-like structures so critical for good nerve functioning are disabled. The excess p-tau then combines to form 'neurofibrillary tangles', which block the neuron's internal transport system, stopping nerves from being able to talk to each other. In terms of predicting brain damage, it's these tangles that are most sinister. Tau, Rachel Buckley tells me, builds up in the hub of the brain and, unlike β-amyloid, 'when it begins to spread, it starts the fundamental changes of Alzheimer's disease as we know it'.

The presence of these β-amyloid and p-tau proteins is recognised by the brain's own immune system as toxic. They stimulate micro-glia from the brain's immune system, which attempt to clear the toxic proteins and other debris from the brain as molecular junk.

But once the microglia are overwhelmed by the task at hand, plaques and tangles start to spread through the cortex of the brain in a pretty predictable pattern and Alzheimer's disease progresses.

But the build-up of toxic β-amyloid and tau proteins doesn't explain everything. Professor Ashley Bush is Head of the Oxidation Biology Unit and Director of the Melbourne Dementia Research Centre, which is a collaboration between Florey Institute of Neuroscience and Mental Health and the University of Melbourne. 'To be honest it's still debatable whether this is the cause of the disorder,' he told me. 'But it is a signature of the brain being in trouble.' This could explain why there are people who die with seemingly perfectly functioning brains but their autopsy reports reveal neurofibrillary tangles and tau. We're not sure why some people are so affected and why others aren't . . . and it's also why treatment directed at β-amyloid and tau protein build-up has been somewhat of a failure.

In terms of symptoms, AD starts with loss of short-term memory (so that a person might ask the same question again and again or keep forgetting appointments), while (at least initially) long-term memory is preserved. The other ability that is affected early in the disease is executive functioning, which involves the performance of complex, goal-oriented tasks along with motivation, strategy development and adjustment, and abstract thinking. All of which are primarily controlled by your prefrontal cortex.

Depression, paranoia, anxiety, apathy and irritability are also often early symptoms although we may not always realise what is going on. These can even appear before memory loss. There are often problems with language (such as trouble remembering common words) and visuospatial dysfunction (which is the inability to recognise faces or common objects).

Later in the disease, we start to see problems with performing complex tasks, and with reasoning and judgement. A good example of this was recently seen in the mother of a friend of mine. Although his mother was a great businesswoman who owned three shops, she uncharacteristically was scammed \$10,000. In hindsight my friend and his siblings realised that his mother was vulnerable to the scam because, due to her developing dementia, she had lost her ability to think straight and use her normal judgement.

Even further down the track, a person might develop difficulty speaking, swallowing and walking. From diagnosis, the disease usually lasts around four to 10 years. Ultimately Alzheimer's disease is fatal. Not everyone realises that.

What the experts do to maintain brain health
PROFESSOR IAN HICKIE

Ian plans on staying in the workforce as long as possible. He eats a Mediterranean diet and drinks a small amount of alcohol with a meal or at social events. He makes sure to manage his sleep by monitoring his circadian rhythm (see Chapter 9 for his tips). He tries to move with purposeful activity and socialises with friends and family members, including his grandchildren. 'I'm not one for supplements,' he told me.

Genes in Alzheimer's disease

About 95 per cent of people with Alzheimer's get it in their mid-60s or older. Getting it at a younger age raises the possibility of a genetic cause. Researchers have studied a number of genes that potentially increase the risk of early onset dementia but have not been able to isolate one which predicts it.

What are genes and how do they work?

Every single cell in your body is made up of a combination of genes and chromosomes. Each cell has 23 different pairs of chromosomes, which are formed out of units of deoxyribonucleic acid (DNA).

A gene is a short section of DNA. Each chromosome has thousands of individual genes.

Genes are passed down from your parents and they carry information that makes you who you are. They can determine things like your body shape and eye colour. But they also control cell functions critical for cell performance and health.

In what is just a jaw-droppingly complicated but extraordinary system, each gene acts like an instruction manual for a cell, telling it how to manufacture a specific protein. These proteins are the workhorses of your cells: doing, making, being. It turns out that the difference between blue and brown pigment in the eye is a difference in proteins made by the cells in the iris of the eye. The difference isn't relevant. But when a gene goes rogue it will give the cell a dud recipe to make a protein that is not quite right.

We know rogue genes are involved in Alzheimer's disease. One in four people have a family history of dementia. And having a family history of dementia doubles your own risk of getting dementia over your lifetime – to 20 per cent.

Genes for late onset Alzheimer's disease

Over 20,000 studies have been published on the genetics of AD so far, and more than 690 rogue genes have been linked with dementia. And researchers are looking for more. But they're all still at investigation stage.

But we *know* for sure about one rogue gene that definitely links to Alzheimer's disease and that's the apolipoprotein E (APOE) gene. The APOE genes are located on chromosome 19, where they provide instructions for making a protein called apolipoprotein E. This protein combines with fats in the body to form molecules called lipoproteins. Lipoproteins package up cholesterol and other fats and carry them through the bloodstream.

Quite what these apolipoprotein E molecules do in the brain is not entirely known but we think they help the microglia clear β-amyloid out of the cells and stop it accumulating. We have tons of research now that tells us that mutations in this gene predisposes you to all forms of dementia, Alzheimer's disease specifically, as well as cardiovascular disease. There are three mutations – or alleles – that we are familiar with: APOE e2, APOE e3, and APOE e4.

The APOE e3 allele is the most common, especially in people of Northern European ancestry, but is less common in people with Asian ancestry. It has no bearing on your dementia risk.

People with the rarer APOE e2 allele tend to have lower LDL (or bad) cholesterol levels but high TG (or triglycerides) and it turns out that this mutation might actually protect you from dementia.

The APOE e4 allele is the one associated with the impairment of the microglial cells' ability to clear excess β-amyloid. This allele has been linked to a higher risk of late onset Alzheimer's disease (AD that develops after the age of 65). It also seems to bring the condition on earlier. People who have inherited one copy of this APOE e4 mutation from one of their parents have a slightly higher dementia risk but people with two copies of APOE e4 genes (one from each parent) have an increased risk of developing Alzheimer's disease and dementia by between five and eight times.

Having said all of this, even with the APOE e4 allele, dementia is *not* inevitable. In fact, most people with APOE e4 will never develop Alzheimer's disease. After all, it's a super common gene; one study found the APOE e4 gene in 24 per cent of the population, and there are also many people with Alzheimer's disease who are APOE e4 negative.

Genes for early onset dementia

Less than 10 per cent of Alzheimer's disease is what we call early onset AD. People with this condition typically get it between their 30s and mid-60s. And in some cases, a genetic mutation is involved.

There are three important mutations we need to discuss that are associated with early onset Alzheimer's disease, but together these only account for between 5 and 10 per cent of early onset dementia. The rest we still don't fully understand.

1. Amyloid precursor protein (APP) on chromosome 21.
2. Presenilin 1 (PSEN1) on chromosome 14.
3. Presenilin 2 (PSEN2) on chromosome 1.

Each of these mutations plays a role in the breaking down of the amyloid precursor protein into the toxic forms of β-amyloid, which eventually leads to the formation of plaques.

Vascular dementia

Vascular dementia, or dementia caused by vascular disease of the brain, accounts for between 5 per cent and 10 per cent of dementia. But autopsy studies show that in 80 per cent of diagnosed Alzheimer's cases in older people, vascular dementia is also present. If these two issues happen together, the dementia is much worse and the progression from mild cognitive impairment to full blown dementia is quicker. This is *really* critical because while trying to prevent and find a cure for Alzheimer's disease has been difficult, vascular dementia *is* largely preventable.

Like other forms of vascular disease, cerebrovascular disease happens when the blood vessels in the brain are damaged by the same sort of atherosclerosis that causes heart disease. This results in brain damage from not receiving enough blood and therefore oxygen or nutrients. But it's when the *small* vessels of the brain are affected by atherosclerosis that we see the highest risk of cognitive impairment and dementia, as opposed to atherosclerosis of larger vessels that appear in places like the neck.

Blockages in the small blood vessels are unlikely to give you the sudden and dramatic strokes that are obvious and devastating to the people who experience them. The onset of a small blockage is more insidious. And there might be *no* signs whatsoever until you start forgetting things and losing that all important executive function and processing speed. But the good news is, there are things we can do to significantly reduce our risk of vascular dementia. And this is why we will spend so much time in this book talking about diet, exercise, getting your blood pressure, body mass index and cholesterol sorted!

> ### What the experts do to maintain brain health
> ### ASSISTANT PROFESSOR RACHEL BUCKLEY
>
> As an APOE carrier herself, taking steps to ward off dementia is critical for Rachel. Her diet of choice? Intermittent fasting. She was drawn in by the longevity data coming out of animal studies and data around famines. 'I've been on the 5:2 for 8 years,' she tells me. Not for weight loss. That's never been an issue for her. Now as a mum of two young girls she simply doesn't eat in daylight hours on Mondays and Thursdays but enjoys a normal dinner. 'I don't want my girls to think I'm dieting,' she tells me. She has totally cut out caffeine, mainly to combat migraines (not really for brain health) but she drinks alcohol. Her supplement of choice? Vitamin D.

Lewy body dementia

Lewy body dementia accounts for 5 per cent of dementia. One of our genes, called the SNCA gene, found on chromosome 4, provides the recipe for making a protein called alpha-synuclein. We don't know exactly what this protein does except that it is abundant in neurons around the synapses, the functioning of which is vital for normal brain function. Scientists have found at least six mutations in the SNCA gene that seem to cause Lewy body dementia. The mutations, or dud recipe, ensure the alpha-synuclein proteins produced have a weird shape and get stuck in the synapses of the brain.

Clumps of abnormal alpha-synuclein are called Lewy bodies. In Lewy body dementia these clumps build up on and around the neurons and cluster around the cerebral cortex.

In many ways the symptoms of Lewy body dementia are similar to those of Alzheimer's disease, but there are typically very early symptoms of sleep disturbances, along with visual hallucinations and visuospatial impairment. These can all happen *before* a person starts experiencing memory impairment.

Frontotemporal lobe degeneration (FTLD)

This is a heartbreaking condition in that it affects the young. About 60 per cent of people with FTLD are aged 45 to 60 years old. Overall, FTLD accounts for 3 per of dementia cases but over 10 per cent of those diagnosed with dementia at age 65 or younger. But we think that that number, which we got from autopsy studies, is likely to be a significant underestimate, as the modern molecular techniques currently used to diagnose FTLD didn't exist when these studies were done.

Some people with FTLD experience major changes in their personality and behaviour with a mixture of apathy and disinhibition. So, they might take their clothes off or be inappropriate and rude to people or even start shoplifting. This personality change is often so severe that family members don't recognise the cognitive decline. Speech is also often affected.

Parkinson's disease dementia

Parkinson's disease dementia (PDD) is defined by changes in thinking and behaviour in someone with a diagnosis of Parkinson's disease (PD). Up to 80 per cent of people with PD eventually develop dementia. The average time between diagnosis of PD and the development of PDD is about 10 years. PD itself is characterised mostly by progressive slowing down of movements, a tremor (at rest), and walking instability, which can cause falls. It is not really known what causes PD in the first place.

The features of PDD are incredibly similar to Lewy body dementia (with sleep issues and hallucinations). But in the latter, movement problems start after the appearance of dementia symptoms and in PDD it's the other way around.

Limbic predominant age-related TDP-43 encephalopathy (LATE)

LATE was only described for the first time in 2019, but experts suspect that it might account for one in five people currently diagnosed with Alzheimer's disease, especially those over 80 years of age, despite the fact that the conditions are so different.

The TARDBP (or TAR DNA binding protein) gene provides the recipe for making a protein called TDP-43 (or transactive response DNA binding protein). In normal situations, TDP-43 sits in the nucleus of a cell, helping mRNA (or messenger RNA) and DNA strands heal themselves, plus carrying out a range of other maintenance jobs. In some cases, a mutation in the gene sees the TDP-43 protein take on a couple of funny shapes (such as when it is phosphorylated, much like p-tau) and that seems to cause it to build up in the cells. Consequently, the cell's DNA is unable to repair itself.

This problem has been found in a stack of neurodegenerative diseases, including 45 per cent of people with frontotemporal dementia. And now we suspect it might be the cause of much of what we have previously been calling Alzheimer's disease. In 2016, groundbreaking research using data from 1000 autopsies found that 50 per cent of people who'd previously been diagnosed with Alzheimer's disease had a build-up of abnormal TDP-43 proteins, often along with the usual Alzheimer's brain features.

Like tau, abnormal forms of TDP-43 initially hit the amygdala before spreading to the hippocampus and eventually the cortex.

If accumulations of these abnormal forms of TDP-43 occur on their own without any β-amyloid or tau, a person's memory is the first to go while other cognitive problems come on later. It seems that the memory loss is more gradual and less severe than in Alzheimer's disease. But if abnormal forms of TDP-43 *plus* β-amyloid and tau are present, a person will develop a more severe dementia than if they had any of the pathologies on their own.

At this point, the condition only shows up on MRI scans when it is severe. And there is no treatment. We need biomarkers (biological molecules found in blood, other body fluids or tissues that can indicate the presence of abnormalities or early stages of disease) for conditions like LATE because if it is a completely separate issue, we should perhaps hold fire on trying drugs that target β-amyloid alone on people with this problem.

I have described these different types of dementia as separate entities, but as you know, they often occur together. Given the appalling lack of treatments, the diagnosis is a 'nice-to-have' but wouldn't change anything. Essentially, we still do not know what is happening in the brains of people with dementia.

What does matter is working on treatments and to develop an effective treatment we really need to have a better understanding of what exactly is happening inside the brain.

Why the brain fails with dementia

Symptoms of dementia occur when nerve cells (neurons) in parts of the brain involved in thinking, learning and memory (cognitive function) have been damaged or destroyed. There is quite a bit of reserve in your brain, so you need to lose a fair chunk of neurons to get failure of the brain.

So what causes this damage to our neurons?

Again, while it is not yet known *exactly* what is happening in our brains with dementia, there is a range of thoughts about what *could* be happening being proposed by current researchers and scientists. And through scientific research we are slowly building a patchwork picture of what is going on inside failing brains.

THE AMYLOID CASCADE HYPOTHESIS

This is the current dominant theory and I have already discussed it a bit in the section on Alzheimer's disease. It is based on observations that clumps of β-amyloid, known as plaques, form outside the cells in our brain. The β-amyloid plaques directly harm the nerves they surround and also trigger a cascade of neuron-killing or neurodegenerative processes that ultimately lead to Alzheimer's disease. As a result, the brain becomes less efficient and then fails to rinse out the toxic β-amyloid, causing more build-up and damage. However, this is still just a hypothesis.

As Professor Bush, Head of the Oxidation Biology Unit and Director of the Melbourne Dementia Research Centre, explained, there is a problem with this hypothesis: plaques have been found in the brains of many elderly people with completely normal cognition.

Melbourne-based practising cognitive neurologist and neuroscientist Dr Trevor Chong adds: 'If you remove amyloid, it should get rid of dementia. We know from all the failed drug trials that it doesn't.'

Bottom line, this is just further proof that our understanding has a long way to go. While this hypothesis hasn't led to successful drug trials, it is still the leading theory.

BLOOD-BRAIN BARRIER ISSUES

We know that the blood vessels in our brain are organised with impressive precision, mirroring the major brain circuits that do the heavy lifting in terms of sensation, memory and motion. Recent studies suggest that changes in the integrity of the blood–brain barrier and deficits in the brain's blood flow happen early on, before any dementia is obvious. The breakdown in the blood–brain barrier has been shown to contribute to neurodegeneration in the brain, perhaps by allowing toxic chemicals to damage the delicate neurons.

THE 'CHOLINERGIC DEFICIT' HYPOTHESIS OF AD

This hypothesis is based on the depleting levels of a key chemical we see in neurons that powers them up. I'm going to give you the simplest explanation I can come up with for this hypothesis, which is essentially that a decrease in acetylcholine causes neuron damage. Acetylcholine was the very first neurotransmitter discovered. It is part of the autonomic nervous system, so it does things like contract the smooth muscles that line blood vessels, dilate blood vessels, increase bodily secretions and slow the heart rate. It is also essential for processing memory and learning. Acetylcholine levels in people with Alzheimer's disease go down and the acetylcholine that is still present in neurons is less effective. This hypothesis has underpinned the earliest drug treatment strategies for Alzheimer's disease.

THE GLUTAMATERGIC HYPOTHESIS

This hypothesis poses the idea that damage to neurons results from damage to the N-methyl-d-aspartate (NMDA) receptors. These are key receptors that are the targets of specific glutamate neurotransmitters on your neurons. These NMDA receptors play an important role in the strengthening of synapses. They're especially important in forming and storing memories. A sudden deactivation of the NMDA receptors can induce psychiatric problems like hallucinations, delusions, agitation, lack of motivation, mood issues and cognitive deficits.

But, as the brain ages, the NMDA receptor system becomes progressively weaker. At the same time, you see excessive compensatory production of the neurotransmitters glutamate and acetylcholine in the brain, which also contribute to degeneration. Boosting NMDA receptor function is now an important theoretical therapeutic strategy to prevent and reverse mild cognitive impairment and dementia.

INFLAMMATION ON THE BRAIN (NEUROINFLAMMATION)

Many scientists believe that dementia might be due to a well-intentioned immune system going rogue with an over-enthusiastic response to the excess β-amyloid and tau. Of course, our cellular systems evolved many hundreds of thousands of years ago. Back then few of us lived long enough to develop dementia as infections, famine or war wiped out most of us. So, our immune system assumes any faulty brain tissue is due to a germ, not dementia.

But sometimes the regulation of this process goes awry. Immune cells called microglial macrophages that are dispersed throughout the brain become increasingly activated as we get older, but much more so when the brain is under stress (such as when a person is experiencing poor diet, lack of sleep, toxins, etc).

The activation of these microglial macrophages means that they produce key pro-inflammatory chemicals. These include interleukin-1β, interleukin-6 (IL-6) and tumour necrosis factor-α (TNF-α). This sets up a cycle of inflammatory processes that culminate in the build up of β-amyloid and eventual neuronal cell death, thinning of the cortex of the brain and reduced brain volume, along with problems with the brain's blood vessels that lead to 'microbleeds' and mini strokes.

Studies have found that people who experience brain fog after COVID-19 also have clear signs of neuroinflammation on an MRI scan. I know, that's a bit concerning. We'll have to wait and see whether getting COVID-19 is a risk for developing dementia earlier.

VASCULAR CASCADE HYPOTHESIS

The idea here is that a combination of bad genes and bad lifestyle results in the blood vessels that supply tiny parts of the brain narrowing. That in turn results in a chronic lack of oxygen to the brain tissues. Dr Allen Orehek is Managing Director and founder of the Dementia Prevention Center in Pennsylvania. He explained that this is happening at micro levels; he has coined the phrase MICRON strokes. He says if you only have one or two a day your brain can compensate, and you'll have no symptoms. But if you have tens or even hundreds every day, you can end up with white matter changes in the brain that can be picked up on an MRI. But by then, the problem is established. 'We're literally missing so much of so many parts of the brain potentially going down the tubes and by the time we pick it up they're so far down the track,' he lamented.

Dr Orehek often checks people for gene mutations which increase their risk of blood clots, such as Factor V Leiden, because these could potentially block off small vessels in the brain, starving it of blood. Early research points to the fact that people with a Factor V Leiden mutation have double the risk of dementia. This mutation, which is found in one in 20–25 Australians, changes a protein in your blood called Factor V and makes you more prone to clotting. So perhaps the clotting is the missing link there.

In truth, it's probably a combination of all of these . . . we still don't know.

What the experts do to maintain brain health
PROFESSOR ALLEN OREHEK

Allen doesn't stick to any specific diet but exercises like a 'fiend', especially Cross Fit and mountain biking. He doesn't take any supplements for brain health but does occasionally and sporadically take vitamin B6, vitamin B12, fish oil and a men's multivitamin for general wellbeing. He has regular check-ups with various specialists to monitor his heart and sleep health (and so far so good!). He doesn't do any brain training but loves his coffee.

It's not just about the chemistry . . .

Dr Michael Sughrue is a co-founder and chief medical officer at Omniscient Neurotechnology, a data company that provides critical information about the brain. Omniscient has researched a variety of brain-related disorders, including depression, chronic pain, brain cancer and bi-polar disorder as well as Alzheimer's and other dementias. Mike might be a business tycoon now but he started out life as a neurosurgeon and he tells me he still thinks like a surgeon. Which means the *location* of the processes above matters just as much as the nature of the process. Because cell death in one part of the brain will look completely different to cell death in another part.

'We've been thinking about dementia as a chemical problem, whereas what they really have is a chemical problem on a circuit board. Where it happens matters,' he told me. 'In neurosurgery we know that doing something wild and crazy in your right frontal lobe might not end in disaster. But doing the same thing in the brainstem sure will!' This explains why dementia can be so different for different people.

Mild cognitive impairment (MCI)

Alzheimer's disease is thought to begin 20 years or more before any symptoms start. There are usually changes happening within the brain that would be visible if you were to have an autopsy, but generally symptoms at this stage are missed altogether by the sufferer.

Mild cognitive impairment (MCI) is the term used to identify those people who are experiencing some memory and other issues, but it is so mild it hasn't yet impaired their ability to perform their usual daily activities. Symptoms of mild cognitive impairment include memory loss, language difficulties, problems with attention and even disorientation. According to different studies, anywhere between 3 per cent and 22 per cent of people over the age of 65 are affected by mild cognitive impairment. Of these people, 5 to 15 per cent progress to dementia every year.

But here's the important thing to know: overall, only 50 per cent of people diagnosed with MCI will progress to Alzheimer's dementia while 15 to 20 per cent will go on to have another type of dementia, but between 35 to 40 per cent will never develop dementia at all. Here is the mega-important bit: we know that the risks for dementia (such as high blood pressure, lack of exercise, poor diet, depression, etc) are the *same* risks for progression from mild cognitive impairment to full blown dementia.

And therein lies the biggest dilemma. The wide variety of symptoms and lack of a clear test result makes diagnosing MCI super tricky. And yet, the damage done to the brain by the time a person develops full blown dementia is so severe that up to this day all treatments have been disappointing. Experts all agree the time to act will be at the MCI stage, so getting a diagnosis early is going to be critical. Eventually.

Signs of MCI to watch out for

This is hard, as people with early cognitive impairment, and even dementia, often don't realise they have an issue. And you may not be able to expect much more from your doctor. In one study set in GP practices, less than 25 per cent of the doctors noted any signs of cognitive issues, even in older people who had what could be described as 'moderate to severe impairment'. Right now, researchers at the Mayo Clinic in Rochester, Minnesota, are conducting research using PET imaging and testing of the cerebrospinal fluid, accessed via a spinal tap, to follow about 3000 people to look at different outcomes. These include how tau and β-amyloid plaques (alone or in combination) have an impact on cognitive function and the development of both mild cognitive impairment and Alzheimer's disease. They have already found subtle but statistically significant differences in the personalities of people with otherwise normal brain function, but whose test results showed evidence of emerging Alzheimer's disease. During the transition to MCI these people had a noticeable decrease in openness, along with signs of physical stress, depression, anxiety and irritability.

In Chapter 3 I'm going to talk about the latest in tests and biomarkers for MCI. Because while midlife is the most important time to act to prevent the development of dementia, early stages of MCI also offer a window to get all your ducks in a row and go all out to halt progression.

Can we treat dementia?

Spoiler alert. Not really.

If depleted acetylcholine levels are one cause of dementia, then developing drugs aimed at restoring acetylcholine levels would be a great thing. *Voila*, cholinesterase inhibitors such as donepezil, rivastigmine and galantamine have been developed.

Cognitive neurologist Dr Trevor Chong prescribes these regularly to patients who can take them (lots of people are on drugs that interact with them) and says they're not a complete failure. 'There is evidence that they can slow decline by about 12 months or so, but the effects are variable between individuals,' he explained. Some people become less aggressive, some people gain small improvements in their memory or their ability to function. 'It's impossible to predict who will benefit or what benefits they'll get,' he says. But he argues it's worth a shot for almost everyone.

If the cholinesterase inhibitors don't work, he often tries his patients on a trial of one of the other group of drugs, the N-methyl-d-aspartate (NMDA) modulators such as memantine, designed to calm down and preserve NMDA receptor activity by tamping down those excessive excitatory glutamate signals.

However, these drugs, don't do much more than the cholinesterase inhibitors, and they can also have numerous side effects such as agitation, urinary incontinence, diarrhoea and insomnia, some of which increase safety concerns.

If the person's family or carers don't notice much change and the person is still declining after six months or so, Dr Chong usually suggests they call the drug a fail and stop.

What the experts do to maintain brain health
DR MICHAEL SUGHRUE

Michael drinks diet Coke and doesn't exercise a lot. He does eat healthily and doesn't drink alcohol or smoke. He doesn't take vitamins but does get regular medical check-ups for his blood pressure and cholesterol.

Future directions

I really feel there are reasons to be optimistic. Perhaps not for people with existing dementia or even mild cognitive impairment, but for those of us at midlife wondering what our futures hold.

New information in the understanding of the mechanisms behind dementia, plus advances in the diagnostics space, has allowed us to take research into combating the disease to the next level.

In 2022, SAGE-718, a new drug in a class of drugs called positive allosteric modulator of N-methyl-D-aspartate (NMDA) receptors, showed some promising results in a two-week trial carried out in 26 patients aged 50–80 years with mild Alzheimer's disease and mild cognitive impairment. The people taking the experimental drug showed improvements in cognition plus executive functioning, learning and memory. Okay so the study only had 26 patients and was not blind – both the researchers and the patients knew what they were getting – that is a long way from a cure. But I am excited about the potential of these new drugs to change the game!

A completely different group of drugs have targeted the β-secretase enzyme that cleaves the amyloid precursor protein into different forms of β-amyloid, including the ultra-toxic β-amyloid 42. It has taken over 20 years to get to the point where a drug can cross the blood–brain barrier and actually switch off β-secretase. In early studies the β-site APP cleaving enzyme 1 (BACE1) inhibitors seem to be able to lower β-amyloid levels in the human brain and in tests involving animals appears to reverse some cognitive decline. In humans, six BACE1 inhibitors have now reached the second and third phases of clinical trials. However, these have had a few hiccups. Contrary to what we expected and hoped for, these drugs didn't just fail; they caused more damage. The people taking them developed worse cognitive function than those on a placebo and they had a reduced brain volume. I think we're all devastated by this. But scientists aren't giving up. Research is ongoing.

You might have already heard of the drug aducanumab, which is a monoclonal antibody against β-amyloid. It was given provisional approval for use in the US despite some major misgivings by neurologists. Trials showed a terrific reduction in brain β-amyloid plaques and β-amyloid-related brain damage. The problem was it was far less impressive when it came to actual changes in the people taking it. The results might have looked stellar on a scan, but it was less impressive in giving people their brains back. Subsequently allegations of fraud threw an even greater shadow over the drug.

I asked Professor Henrik Zetterberg about the aducanumab controversy. He is Professor of Neurochemistry at the University of Gothenburg in Sweden. Like me, he is actually optimistic about this kind of drug. He just thinks people may need to start taking it earlier to obtain meaningful changes. People with established dementia often have so much physical disease in their brains it can be hard to regrow enough brain tissue to change outcomes, even after removing lots of β-amyloid. 'When you have someone with symptoms of Alzheimer's disease, half the hippocampi are gone and the other half are full of amyloid,' he explained.

The challenge is to understand dementia better to target the right drug to the right person at the right stage of the disease. Professor Zetterberg's research into biomarkers will hopefully enable us to do just that.

But in the meantime, it's all about prevention. And that's why I wrote this book. To give you the tools to make the best decisions regarding your brain health.

Takeaways

- There is a difference between an ageing brain and one that is developing dementia. However, the symptoms can overlap.
- If you mislay your keys, that is not a cause for concern that you have dementia. If you don't know what to do with your keys when you find them, that is when you need to start worrying.
- Only 50 per cent of people diagnosed with MCI will progress to Alzheimer's dementia.
- The best time to start preventing the onset of MCI and dementia is in midlife.
- The risks factors between developing MCI and then MCI progressing to full blown dementia are the same. Looking after sleep, diet and lifestyle can prevent both the development of MCI and then progression of MCI to dementia.

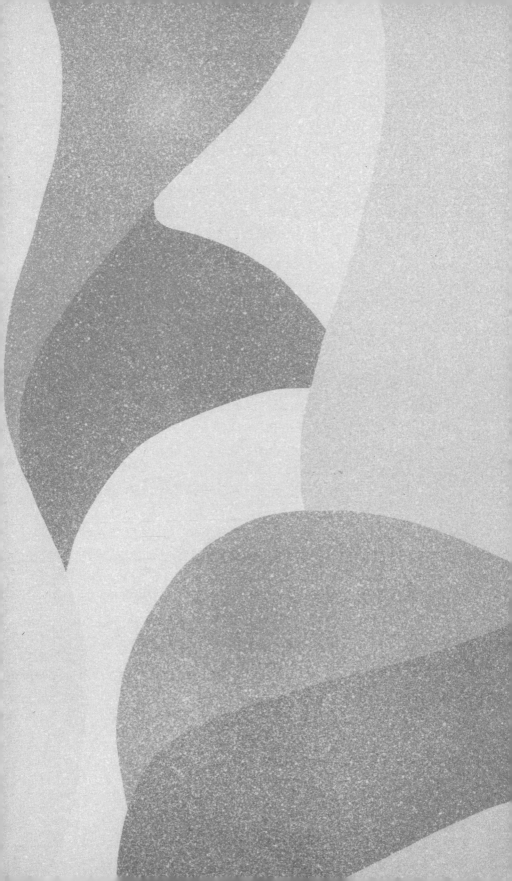

CHAPTER 3

Help, I keep losing my keys! Am I getting dementia?

I probably don't go a day without someone sharing with me their concerns about their brains, such as lately they can't remember things; they forgot the name of someone they knew for years – it was so embarrassing! They lose their keys/phone/umbrella or sunglasses. They double-booked a coffee catch-up and then did it again the following week. What is going on? They ask for a test for dementia. Or more particularly, they ask, is dementia on its way? Can it be picked up now before it really kicks in?

As we have already discussed in Chapter 2, there has been a huge amount of research already focused on detecting signs of early dementia or mild cognitive impairment so we can take evasive action before too much brain cell damage has happened. Here I have pretty grim news to report. Despite the mountains of research, scientists still have no good predictor of who will develop dementia, especially Alzheimer's disease.

Diagnosing dementia

Of the estimated 55 million people living with dementia around the world, only one in four have been formally diagnosed with the condition. In 2021, Alzheimer's Disease International released their World Alzheimer Report. 'Key barriers to diagnosis identified by people with dementia and carers included lack of access to trained clinicians (47 per cent), fear of diagnosis (46 per cent) and cost (34 per cent),' the authors stated. The experts surveyed blamed a lack of access to specialised diagnostic tests (38 per cent), a lack of knowledge in making a diagnosis (37 per cent) and the belief that nothing could be done (33 per cent, i.e. believing there is no point in getting a diagnosis) as barriers to diagnosis.

Despite this, there is a huge and growing focus on getting that timely diagnosis because this will allow people with dementia and their families to do whatever they can to slow the inevitable cognitive loss and maintain quality of life.

Unlike a tumour in the body or a stomach ulcer, getting a biopsy of brain tissue and looking at it under a microscope is close to impossible. We'd have to bore through the skull to get a sample, and in the process could do some major damage. The person having this done would also need a stint in hospital. So, dementia is normally diagnosed by testing cognitive functions, especially memory. If these tests indicate possible problems, we then use a stack of other tests such as blood tests and scans like a CT scan or MRI. Together they help to rule out other causes of the symptoms, such as a brain tumour, thyroid problems or a urine infection. But these tests are notoriously inaccurate. As Dr Michael Sughrue, co-founder of Omniscient Neurotechnology, a company involved in research into a variety of brain-related disorders including dementias, describes: 'We have these measuring sticks that are overly blunt.'

They sure are! They often remain negative until the person has severe or even end-stage dementia.

Cognitive assessments

These are tests administered by a GP, an occupational therapist, psychologist or a nurse to check your mental abilities, such as memory or thinking.

On the next few pages I have listed some tests that can be done by a professional or even yourself if you do a bit of reading about how to do them. The updated UK dementia guidelines found most of these cognitive assessment tools to be pretty similar in their accuracy, so you only need to pick one.

None of these tests formally diagnose dementia or even mild

cognitive impairment. They need follow-up with a doctor. They're just screening tests to tell you if further investigations might be needed.

As an example of how inaccurate and variable the testing for dementia can be, I keep thinking about one of my patients, who, at least to me, was obviously suffering from dementia. She lived alone and I was really worried about her. She came to me because she wanted clearance to renew her driver's licence. I ran her through the 30-point Mini-Mental State Exam (see below), which is the current screen GPs are advised to use, then sent her off to the psychogeriatrician at our local teaching hospital for a formal diagnosis. To my dismay, her report came back clear. This happened for several years in a row, until one day she had a fall, ended up in hospital and community services became involved. And it was in hospital, with access to better testing, that she was finally diagnosed with dementia. I had several calls from the social workers and her daughters asking me why she hadn't been tapped into dementia services earlier. I had to explain that the experts had always declared her fit and well and, in fact, only three weeks before had written to me saying she didn't have dementia! And just nine weeks after she got the psychogeriatrician all clear and six weeks after her fall, she was in a dementia care nursing home.

The Mini-Mental State Examination (MMSE)

Dr Marshal Folstein first developed this test in 1975. Since then, it has become one of the most common screening tests for cognitive impairment and it is routinely used to rule people in and out of clinical trials. It's also super commonly used by GPs and nurses and takes about 10 minutes. A person is asked a series of questions to test both their memory and, to a much lesser extent, their executive function. The maximum score for the MMSE is 30. A score of 25 out of 30 or higher is normal, while a score below 24 is considered abnormal, indicating possible cognitive impairment. It's an older test and there are probably better tests around. That doesn't stop it from being the test GPs are advised to administer when doing screening in practice.

The General Practitioner Assessment of Cognition (GPCOG)

This is a screening tool for cognitive impairment designed for use in primary care. There is an option for the 'informant' to do the test, so you can do the test online *for* someone, such as your parent, by heading to http://gpcog.com.au even if they won't come with you. It is super quick and easy.

The Memory Impairment Screen

This is another screen that is a four-minute, four-item memory test. It's best conducted by an expert who has experience administering a test like this, but if you're interested, you can check it out at https://www.alz.org/media/Documents/memory-impairment-screening-mis.pdf

The Mini-Cog

This is a three-minute evaluation consisting of a recall exercise for memory and a scored clock-drawing test. It can't be done at home and needs to be done in person (not via Telehealth). It can be used effectively after brief training and results must be evaluated by a health provider to determine if a full-diagnostic assessment is needed. It can't provide a diagnosis.

The Addenbrooke's Cognitive Examination-Revised (ACE-R)

This test was originally developed to flesh out the MMSE. It tests five separate cognitive domains: attention/orientation, memory, language, verbal fluency and visuospatial skill, with a score out of 100. Scores below 64 are pretty accurate for diagnosing dementia. Scores between 65 and 69 suggest MCI, but that is less accurate. It takes about 20–25 minutes to do.

The Eight-item Informant Interview to Differentiate Aging and Dementia (AD8)

This is an eight-question interview used to tell the difference between a person who is simply getting older or has mild dementia. This tool looks at changes over time and can be administered at home and then taken to the GP. It can be found at https://www.alz.org/media/Documents/ad8-dementia-screening.pdf

The Short Informant Questionnaire on Cognitive Decline in the Elderly (IQCODE)

This is a screening tool that evaluates cognitive decline and dementia in a loved one. There are 16 online questions and it takes about five minutes to do. It has been described as a moderately effective test with accuracy rates of between 60 and 74 per cent in studies. This test could be administered at home by a carer or relative and then taken to the GP for the next steps. It is found at https://www.alz.org/media/documents/short-form-informant-questionnaire-decline.pdf

The Montreal Cognitive Assessment (MoCA)

This is a 10–15 minute, 30-question test. A score of 26 or more determines a person's cognitive state as normal. It is more accurate than the MMSE, especially in people with higher levels of education.

Which test should be done?

A 2015 review found that the Mini-Cog test and the ACE-R came up trumps for diagnosing dementia, while the MoCA was best for diagnosing mild cognitive impairment. All results must be checked out by a health provider to determine if a full-diagnostic assessment is needed as the tests can't really provide a clinical diagnosis.

Who should be evaluated for cognitive impairment?

Anyone with memory concerns or other cognitive complaints should be assessed. But it's not just memory issues that might indicate some cognitive impairment. There are other triggers like personality changes, new depression, deterioration of a chronic disease without explanation, and falls or balance issues. Often the person themself has zero interest in being assessed, telling you they're fine and it's your issue. I see this all the time and it can be really hard to get someone to accept the need for an assessment.

But once a test has picked up an issue and, to be honest, even if it's normal but there's a compelling story of personality changes, short-term memory issues or problems with executive function, it's time for a trip to the doctor.

Additional tests done by your doctor

If we are thinking about a diagnosis of dementia or mild cognitive impairment, a GP will do a physical examination to pick up any signs that might indicate a neurological problem. We also need to check for visual or auditory problems that can make every-thing worse. We'd also run a batch of blood tests. Routine blood tests help to rule out conditions like diabetes or high cholesterol which can contribute to vascular dementia alone or which can make Alzheimer's disease worse. We can also rule out liver or kidney failure, or any vitamin deficiencies, that can also worsen cognitive performance. We would then potentially do a chest

X-ray and ECG, depending on risk factors and the previous test results.

Scans

Scans are an awesome tool for monitoring progression of dementia and even mild cognitive impairment. When it comes to scans, we break them into two groups. Anatomic imaging refers to computed tomography (CT) and magnetic resonance imaging (MRI). (MRI also refers to ultrasound and X-ray but they're not used for the brain.) Metabolic brain imaging refers to [18F]-fluorodeoxyglucose (18F-FDG) positron emission tomography, better known as PET scans.

At this stage everything you're about to read is about diagnosing someone to confirm a diagnosis of dementia. Scans are not a predictor of future cognitive decline.

Anatomical imaging

These days scans allow you to just lie on a table fully clothed and a scanner can see inside your brain. The images are then collated using sophisticated software to create highly accurate 3D images of your brain without the need for neurosurgery. Sometimes certain dyes are injected into your veins to enhance the quality of the images further.

MRI scans

The peak international body, Alzheimer's Disease International, recently recommended that magnetic resonance imaging (MRI) or computed tomography (CT) of the brain should be considered as part of the initial evaluation of dementia in everyone.

These scans are done both to confirm the brain looks like a brain with dementia (essentially looking for evidence of brain shrinkage, especially in the hippocampus) and to rule out another cause for the cognitive decline, such as a brain tumour, infection or a stroke.

While a head CT is good to rule out a cancer or diagnose a stroke, and even to assess hippocampal shrinkage, MRIs are better. An MRI can pick up evidence of smaller strokes, as well as small vessel disease, and are better for looking at brain tumours and any shrinkage of the hippocampus. But MRIs are expensive and it can be hard to get one in poorly resourced areas, such as rural and remote districts.

A brain MRI takes around 20 minutes. Sometimes a contrast agent or dye called gadolinium (a rare earth element) is given via the vein to help the radiologists see the brain structures more clearly.

Functional scans

These are scans that look at how the brain is functioning in specific areas. Anatomical scans that look at the structure of the brain are great but if we can combine the ability to discover what's there with what the brain is actually *doing*, we have taken scanning to the next level. This is where functional scans come in. New technology has allowed scientists to measure how actively various parts of the brain respond to different challenges and stimuli.

Functional MRI

Invented in 1990, functional magnetic resonance imaging (fMRI) takes the same MRI scan that looks at the brain's structure but adds a software program to measure tiny changes in blood flow and metabolic changes in brain activity. It is used to measure the parts of the brain performing specific functions. When a specific part of the brain is activated by a task – such as finger tapping on your right hand – the localised brain activation results in increased energy requirement (and therefore oxygen and glucose uptake) in the specifically related brain parts. That increased oxygen or sugar can be seen on the fMRI.

We're still working out how to use fMRI to diagnose dementia, let along mild cognitive impairment or the signs it might be coming.

However, we're not there yet! As a result, it's not the sort of scan that is being ordered by neurologists to diagnose dementia. Rather it is being used in scientific trials and as we get closer to understanding the optimum way to use these scans and as we refine the techniques, eventually they will extend beyond the labs and into a standard radiologist's clinic.

Nuclear medicine scans

A positron emission tomography (PET) scan is a type of nuclear imaging test that uses a radioactive substance and a special camera to create 3D pictures. It can measure the concentration of glucose in regions of the brain to show how different parts are using energy and then use this information to create an image. SPECT scans are nuclear medicine scans that use a slightly different radioactive substance to PET scans. With these targeted scans, you can actually see both β-amyloid and tau in the brain.

In people with dementia, it's not a bad test, although far from perfect. In studies, PET scans have been found to have a sensitivity of 80 per cent (so if 100 people with dementia have a PET scan 80 will be picked up) and a specificity of 70 per cent (so if 100 people have a scan that tells them they have dementia, only 70 per cent actually have it). That is not exactly awesome.

They also expose you to radiation, are horrifically expensive (here in Australia they cost about a thousand dollars a scan) and are really hard to get because not many places do them or have the doctors to interpret them. Although, as clinicians improve their skills and the cost comes down, they'll probably be used more in the future.

Cerebrospinal fluid sampling

Remember the cerebrospinal fluid or CSF? It's the clear fluid that protects, nourishes and clears waste from the brain and spinal cord. Every day, the brain produces nearly half a litre of cerebrospinal fluid, and it contains some important biomarkers that we can look at to diagnose dementia. As previously described, biomarkers are biological molecules found in blood, other body fluids or tissues that indicate any abnormal process or stages of disease. Looking for biomarkers in CSF has some major advantages.

As we know from Chapter 2, β-amyloid plaques are formed from β-amyloid, and the most toxic form of these plaques is β-amyloid 42. We can look at β-amyloid, and specifically at β-amyloid 42 levels, in the CSF directly. In people with Alzheimer's, because the β-amyloid accumulates in the brain instead of being effectively washed, CSF levels are only half the levels of a healthy person. Measuring CSF β-amyloid 42 has a sensitivity of 90 per cent, which means that if 100 people with Alzheimer's disease have this test, 90 per cent will be diagnosed. More importantly CSF levels will start to rise *before* you develop any cognitive symptoms at all.

Tau can also be measured in the CSF. As we know, high levels of both phosphorylated tau (p-tau) and total tau (t-tau) are features of Alzheimer's disease, especially advanced disease. These CSF findings are already there in people with MCI. In fact, CSF β-amyloid 42 levels start to drop off from 20 to 25 years of age and CSF tau increases 20 years before dementia appears. However, experts argue that *at the moment*, they are better for ruling out MCI than ruling it in.

So why don't we just look at everyone's CSF? Because it's super tricky. Firstly, to get your hands on the fluid, you need to have a lumbar puncture (AKA spinal tap), which is not only pretty unpleasant but is also a complex procedure to perform and usually needs to be done in a big teaching hospital by a specialist. Secondly, handling of CSF samples requires some degree of expertise, often with a sophisticated lab and these labs are already completely overworked. It's just not practical.

Plus, what do you do with the information? You now know you have dementia of some sort. What next? Given the grim prognosis and complete absence of evidence-based treatments, it can be a lot of stress for not much upside. As a result, these biomarker tests are limited to unusual cases, such as early onset dementia or in situations where there is rapid progression.

Dr Raymond Schwartz is a practising neurologist and Clinical Associate Professor at the University of Sydney. He tells me that while he has been sending more patients for these CSF tests lately as part of recruitment into clinical trials, he doesn't refer his patients for these tests that often.

What the experts do to maintain brain health
DR RAYMOND SCHWARTZ

Raymond exercises five plus days a week at high intensity for at least 40 minutes at a time. He also practises yoga and mindfulness. He does ocean swimming without a wetsuit as a mindfulness practice. He describes his diet as 'as close to Mediterranean as possible' but admits 'my vice is chocolate'. Another vice is working too much. He believes passionately in a work–life balance but is not quite there yet himself. He takes his cardiovascular risks seriously and gets regular check-ups. 'I think there's a role for natural therapies for cerebrovascular health,' he told me. But he doesn't take any supplements himself.

Blood tests for dementia

If doing a test of CSF is so difficult, what about a simple blood or plasma (the liquid of the blood minus the red blood cells) test to detect biomarkers that could indicate a problem? This is the new frontier I am most excited about.

Scientists such as Professor Ashley Bush from the Florey Institute are examining plasma levels of phosphorylated tau or p-tau in

Alzheimer's disease. 'They reflect the amount of β-amyloid that's accumulating in the brain,' he said. 'We're not yet at the point of having a blood marker that is able to detect the tangles in the brain, but it's relatively early days for that.'

These tests are not commercially available yet but to find out more I spoke to Henrik Zetterberg, Professor of Neurochemistry at the University of Gothenburg in Sweden. With a background in both molecular biology and medicine, Henrik has spent the past 15 years focusing on the development of biomarkers for Alzheimer's disease and other brain disorders. 'The difficulty has been that the concentrations of these biomarkers are so low in blood,' he said. In fact, they are 100 to 1000 times more concentrated in CSF than blood. But advances have meant that we are now seeing the ability to detect even micro fragments of these biomarkers in blood. 'We are quite certain about plasma phospho-tau levels in the blood,' he told me. And these levels correlate well with what is going on in the brain.

> What the experts do to maintain brain health
> ## PROFESSOR HENRIK ZETTERBERG
>
> This is personal for Henrik, whose father has dementia. He is actually a bit fatalistic about dementia and has been fairly reticent to overhaul his (admittedly fairly healthy) lifestyle for the sole purposes of protecting his brain. 'I almost think what happens, happens, and you take it as it comes!' he says.
>
> While it looks like lifestyle interventions make a difference to your chances of getting dementia, Henrik is more excited about pharmacological treatments to prevent worsening cognitive impairment. 'I would like to change the way we deal with Alzheimer's disease but until we achieve this, I have decided not to worry about it,' he told me.

'This is a good situation to be in now because it means that we can find the pathological processes in blood tests and we can work with the pharma industry,' Henrik explained. It gives pharma companies ways of measuring improvements in experimental drugs without having to wait for clunky and often only partially accurate clinical tests or scans. Henrik feels certain that this will deliver meaningful treatments to people who – until now – have had very little hope.

So, can you diagnose brain issues before you even see dementia?

Let's look at some of the science that we are turning to in order to detect issues in the brain before dementia sets in.

Diagnosing mild cognitive impairment

This is *much* harder than diagnosing full blown dementia and we often get it wrong. In fact, studies have shown that the false positive rate for diagnosis of mild cognitive impairment is around 30 per cent. In other words, almost a third of people who are diagnosed with MCI don't have it. Oops. Without any validated test, mild cognitive impairment is a clinical diagnosis – in reality it's the doctor's best professional judgement.

And don't forget, only 50 per cent of people diagnosed with MCI will progress to Alzheimer's or dementia.

Gene screens

Remember how we talked about the genes that contribute to Alzheimer's disease? As a quick reminder, having the APOE e4 allele seems to impair the microglial cells' ability to clear excess β-amyloid and the especially toxic form β-amyloid 42. Having the APOE e4 allele increases your risk of dementia and seems to bring the condition on earlier than might have happened without the gene. People who have one copy of this APOE e4 mutation have a slightly higher dementia risk but people with two copies of APOE e4 genes have an increased risk of developing Alzheimer's disease and dementia by between five and eight times.

Professor Henrik Zetterberg says: 'If you have a parent with Alzheimer's disease, you have a bit of a higher risk. If you have several family members with it, then there is quite a strong risk that is an APOE e4 effect.'

You can find out if you have this gene. Lots of my patients have asked me for these tests. It would be easy enough to do. A blood test can easily identify which APOE alleles you have for example. But that won't help identify whether you will or won't get Alzheimer's disease. After all, 24 per cent of people seem to carry at least one of the APOE e4 allele. And it wouldn't change the advice about how to live your life now to reduce your risk of developing dementia. Nothing would change. For now.

I asked Professor Henrik Zetterberg about this. His father has Alzheimer's disease and with his family history he suspects he is at higher risk of getting the disease himself. 'You could think about a future scenario when you have an established intervention that you know will help and then I would recommend a polygenic risk score, and if you found out you were at high risk then you could go and check your blood biomarkers every second year. And when they start to become abnormal you could do this intervention,' he said. 'And I hope Alzheimer's disease will become such a disease.' But right now, it isn't. We don't have a drug or a procedure that can slow things down any more than just the lifestyle changes and health care we recommend in general. Which is why gene screening isn't a test we offer in general practice. Currently, APOE testing is used more in research settings to identify study participants with a higher risk of developing Alzheimer's and monitor them over time or do certain interventions. Research hasn't come up with a compelling case to test members of the general population who request it. It could just contribute to possibly unnecessary distress, given that it is not a certainty that Alzheimer's will actually develop.

But the future is bright. The rate of new developments, thanks to amazing biotechnology and brilliant scientists, means that the possibility of seeing drugs and interventions that can either stop or at least help the progression of dementias in our lifetime is not that far-fetched!

Takeaways

- Anyone with memory concerns or other cognitive complaints should be assessed. Other incidents like personality changes, new onset of depression, deterioration of a chronic disease without explanation, and falls or balance issues can also be triggers for getting an assessment.
- Testing for Alzheimer's and other dementia-related disorders is mainly done through cognitive tests, followed by MRI or PET scans.
- Testing is still notoriously complicated, as some tests are more accurate than others and not all tests are accessible to everyone, depending on where they live.
- Although tests such as MRI scans and gene testing can detect the presence of dementia precursors, they can't predict the progression of MCI, or MCI towards dementia.

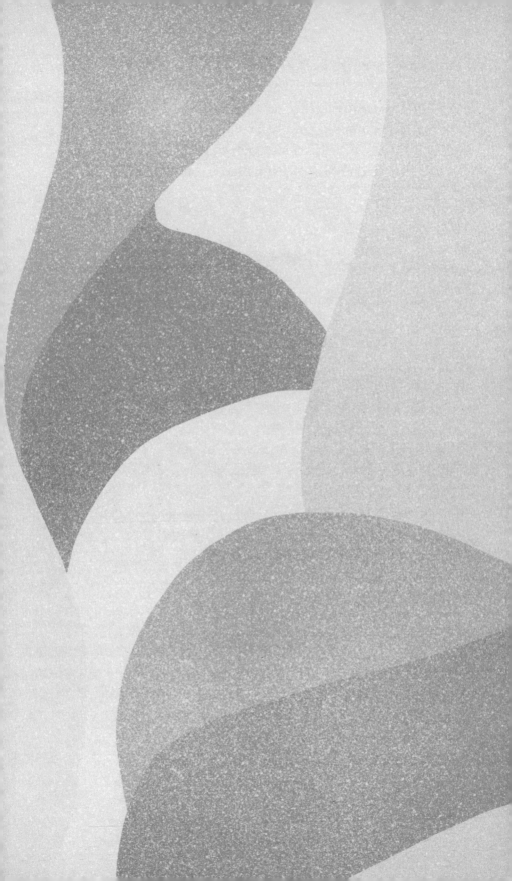

CHAPTER 4

Will exercise help you avoid dementia?

W ithout exception, every expert I spoke to while writing this book was doing some sort of physical exercise to protect their brain. To be honest, it was the only thing everyone agreed on. This is not great news for me, personally. I put exercise of the sweaty-fast moving-virtuous type in the 'developing this skill' column on my personal report card.

Fantasy me goes for a relaxing run or does a spot of yoga most days. Reality me guiltily sits at the computer and feels like a sloth. Being in perimenopause (or peri), I don't love the effects of exercise on my bladder or on my sweat glands. I really envy those people who look effortlessly cool while running. I look like a wilting, soggy, frizzy-haired tomato.

So, I sheepishly admit I was a bit excited to chat to Professor Victor Henderson, Professor of Neurology and Neurological Sciences at Stanford University and Director of the NIH Stanford Alzheimer's Disease Research Center, about exercise and the brain. He insists that finding solid evidence that regular exercise helps to prevent dementia or MCI has its challenges.

'All of us think we should be into fitness and feel guilty if we're not exercising,' he said. But when it comes to exercise, is there any real evidence it works? 'Well, for a certain kind of mouse we know that it does,' he said. 'But while people who exercise develop less dementia, it's not clear that exercise is the cause. That's because the people who exercise are usually the people who do other healthy things too.'

Take the Finnish Geriatric Intervention to Prevent Cognitive Impairment and Disability (FINGER) study, for example. FINGER is a multi-centre randomised controlled trial currently taking place in Finland and 40 other countries including Australia, of people between 60 and 77 years of age who have a higher risk of dementia. The point of this study is to test whether a battery of intervention strategies, including physical exercise *teamed with* nutritional advice, cognitive training, social activities and management of vascular and metabolic risk factors like diabetes, high blood pressure or cholesterol, impact the risk of dementia. One group of people are receiving no interventions whatsoever: they're the control group. For the rest of the people in the study, in addition to the social, dietary and health interventions, they are also participating in a muscle strength training and aerobic exercise program, plus postural balance boosting exercises.

After two years, the study has found that those in the intervention group already have 25 per cent higher performance on cognition scores, 150 per cent higher processing speed, 83 per cent higher executive function scores, 40 per cent better memory and 60 per cent less chronic diseases other than dementia. But can we attribute these amazing gains to the exercise? Not really, according to Professor Henderson. Extended follow-up of the study participants is ongoing. But even then, attributing the benefits to any particular intervention will be a tall order. The reason for this is that there are so many 'variables' in the mix and as Professor Henderson points out, exercisers tend to be generally healthier. For someone who doesn't get dementia, can we say it was the exercise that helped? What if it was their terrific diet or not smoking or drinking to excess? What if they had great blood pressure and no diabetes? Maybe they were never going to get dementia anyway?

Professor Henderson agreed that being sedentary in older age is linked to cognitive impairment, but he is adamant that there's no clear evidence of the relationship being causal. 'A little bit of apathy [about exercise] may represent early signs of cognitive decline,' he points out. I sure hope not! Having made a convincing argument for my self-flagellation over being an exerciser by aspiration only, I asked Professor Henderson about his own habits. It turns out that he does a combination of aerobic and resistance exercise between two and four times a week, and he's in his late 70s. Because while there's no convincing evidence from trials, he's still convinced that regular exercise is a wise move for his health in general, including his brain.

I'm hardly surprised. Professor Ian Hickie is emphatic that regular exercise is a critical tool in preserving your brain health. 'As you age you have to be *more* physically active!' he said. 'You have to push yourself harder, despite the pain in your knees or your back.'

Professor Hickie pointed me in the direction of research that lays out the science behind the benefits of exercise on the brain in a fairly convincing way.

What the experts do to maintain brain health
PROFESSOR VICTOR HENDERSON

Victor does a combination of aerobic and resistance exercise between two and four times a week. He only drinks minimal alcohol – two standard drinks a week. But he loves his coffee and will have four to five a day. Half of those are caffeinated and half decaf. He does not struggle to sleep. He is naturally good at it!

He takes no supplements. Aged in his 70s he is still working at a university, which he says is a very social place to work. It keeps his mind busy.

'I like reading,' he told me. 'I prefer that to watching late night TV shows and the ads for supplements that won't help.'

The case for exercise

In 2003, researchers conducted a meta-analysis of all 18 of the trials done between 1966 and 2001 on various forms of exercise and the consequent impacts on cognition. 'Fitness training was found to have robust but selective benefits for cognition, with the largest fitness-induced benefits occurring for executive-control processes,' the researchers concluded. In other words, fitness training mostly benefits our executive functioning abilities. But the science quality was far from conclusive. The studies were all different: different lengths of time, different levels of ability of the subjects, different exercises done at different intensities. But yes, I have to admit all of these imperfect studies pooled together does suggest that exercise is beneficial in some way for cognitive health.

Then in 2020, Taiwanese and US researchers conducted another meta-analysis looking at subsequent studies done after the last 2003 review. They found 33 newer studies altogether. The studies looked at everything from aerobic to resistance exercise, Tai Chi and yoga, to dance and even coordination exercises. The results concluded that most forms of exercise had some benefits on executive function regardless of how often, how intense, what type, the session time and length. This was true regardless of gender and for all age groups except those over 75 years of age. Caveat: the benefits were described as small.

In 2021, a US study of 180 people aged between 60 and 79 was published. The people were enrolled in a six-month program of either aerobic walking, social dance or a control group of no exercise. All the participants had MRI scans of their brains before and after the exercise program (or in the case of the control group, sitting on the proverbial couch). The exercisers showed signs of improvement on their MRIs while the people who didn't do any exercise saw their MRI results get worse. Interestingly, the walkers *also* had improvements in their performance in some memory tests, but not the dancers. Lastly, improvements in overall fitness did not correlate with changes in the

MRI. Or in other words, the level of fitness a person had did not have any bearing on the results of their MRI.

I find those studies a bit unconvincing. Small gains, in only certain specific exercises. But given that we know doing some kind of regular exercise, at any age, has numerous benefits for your longevity, sleep, mental health, cardiovascular health, blood pressure and risk of diabetes, all of which can impact your brain health, there's probably no excuse to avoid it.

The good news is that if you don't fancy donning your hot pants and doing a formal exercise class, you don't need to despair. Exercise comes in all shapes and sizes.

Gardening

Professor Dimity Pond is Professor of General Practice, Discipline of General Practice, at the University of Newcastle. She is also the author of a number of guidelines around dementia identification and management in general practice. She pointed me to the results of the Dubbo Study of the Elderly, conducted in 2006. This was a prospective study of 2805 men and women aged 60 years and older living in the community and initially free of cognitive impairment. They were first assessed in 1988 and followed for 16 years. This is now my favourite study in the world. Check out these results: any intake of alcohol in this study predicted a 34 per cent *lower* risk of dementia, and while daily walking predicted a 38 per cent lower risk of dementia in men, there was no significant benefit in women. Works for me because I love wine and hate exercise. But back to the gardening bit. It won the exercise game! Daily gardening presented a 36 per cent lower risk of dementia over the 16-year period. It also reduced the risk of ending up in a nursing home.

It could be the exposure to what we call green space. Researchers who were looking at the effects of ginkgo biloba on brain health (which is discussed more fully in the next chapter) also looked at where the people in the study lived in relation to their access to green space and nature. And that access to nature definitely helped delay cognitive deterioration. Having said that, people who lived in houses with a nice garden tend to be in a different socio-economic bracket to those who live in dense urban settings, which could have played a factor in the results. The researchers in the Dubbo study also considered this but still found benefits from exposure to greenery, regardless of financial status.

What the experts do to maintain brain health
PROFESSOR DIMITY POND

'I've walked half an hour a day, five days a week, for the past 10 years,' says Dimity. She admits her weight is a constant battle, but she's never given up trying to keep it under control and sticks to a generally healthy diet. She is a passionate gardener, pointing to the Dubbo Study of the elderly, which favoured gardening over other exercise. She has a book club as well as regular catch-ups with friends and credits her grandchildren with challenging her brain regularly. Dimity has just one coffee a day, then switches to tea out of preference. She takes fish oil supplements for her joints, not her brain, and vitamin D for her bones, but no specific brain supplements. 'I don't have time for brain exercises,' she tells me. As an academic supervising PhD and undergraduate students, she figures she's got that side sorted out!

Tai Chi

I first became fascinated by Tai Chi when I was sent as a young reporter for the *Medical Observer*, an industry newspaper for doctors, to interview Tai Chi master and then GP Dr Paul Lam. I don't know how old he is now, but he was no spring chicken then and yet was light as a feather on his feet with incredible strength and agility, not to mention balance.

Movements in Tai Chi are never forced; the muscles are relaxed rather than tensed, and the joints are never fully extended or bent. There's evidence this form of martial art has benefits for muscle strength, balance, flexibility, osteoporosis, diabetes and arthritis. But a Chinese randomised prospective study in 2013 showed it helped with dementia as well. One hundred and twenty older but independent adults were randomised to either three weekly sessions of Tai Chi, walking, a social get-together, or nothing. After 40 weeks, the Tai Chi group and the social interaction group participants showed significant increases in total brain volume on MRI scanning, as well as improvements on several neuropsychological measures. No statistically significant changes in either assessment were seen in the walking group or the group who did nothing. Interestingly, though, faster walkers had better scores on some cognitive tests than the slower walkers.

Lots of people do Tai Chi outdoors in a park. It looks so beautiful and so serene, and so I have moved learning Tai Chi to number one on the list of other sorts of beneficial exercise.

Grab your mop!

A 2021 study out of Singapore found that older people who did light housework such as washing the dishes, dusting, making the bed, doing or hanging out the laundry, ironing and cooking meals, had better attention and memory. Possibly because housework is reasonably rigorous exercise.

So if the gym is not for you, you can rest assured that doing household chores, such as cleaning the bathroom, will also count towards improving your memory and attention abilities . . . without the cost of any gym fees!

Zero to hero – small steps please!

If you do want to take up exercise, be smart about it. There is no point going from couch to marathon in a month. Start off slowly and try to make meaningful progress every few days to few weeks. We don't have an end point here. But the exercise activity has to be sustainable and reasonably enjoyable, so you don't give it up at the first hurdle.

This might mean roping in a friend to do the activity with you, or doing something a bit out of the ordinary like joining a local tango club or listening to a Spotify playlist that gets you dancing. Try to be mindful on the journey. How does the activity make you feel? More energetic? More relaxed? Are you sleeping better? Look for and bank the benefits as a way of keeping going.

I really love hiking and I try to include a 15 to 25 km hike at least once a year. I know it will be a bit tough so I need to prepare for it. That is my motivation for doing regular training. And it certainly helps me sleep a bit better.

My husband Daniel, on the other hand, is a phenomenal athlete and he does an hour of high-intensity exercise every day, either cycling or running. He also does push-ups and other body-weight exercise regularly. He uses exercise to help his mental as well as his physical health.

Cognitive training

We used to think that you got the brain you got, and it grew until adulthood and then started to age and pare back. It's still true that the basic structure of your brain is determined by your genes. But we now know the brain is constantly on the move, creating new connections, and re-wiring itself to change the way it works to adapt to our ever-changing needs. This is called neuroplasticity and is described in an article called 'The impact of studying brain plasticity' as 'the ability of the nervous system to change its activity in response to intrinsic or extrinsic stimuli by reorganising its structure, functions, or connections'. It is fundamental to the development and function of the brain, and it is essential for learning and memory. It's also the way the brain heals itself after an injury.

And we now also know that we can do things to increase neuro-plasticity. This has created a multibillion-dollar industry of 'brain training games' which claim to have scientific proof that they make your brain younger. This can be such a confusing area. Should you believe the claims and if so, which ones?

The picture for brain or cognitive training is super complex. That's partly because the term 'neuroplasticity' is not a scientific one but rather a blanket term that encompasses a lot of different things. This makes studying it and documenting any improvements from it really hard.

However we define mental activity, it's all good for the brain. For example, studies show that doing cognitively stimulating activities in later life, like reading, playing puzzles and going to museums and concerts, is linked to a lower risk of dementia. Similarly, more challenging or complex careers have been associated with a lower risk of dementia in later life.

But do the benefits of having an active brain from visiting a museum or staying in the workforce also extend to playing an online game or doing other 'cognitive training'?

Brain games

There is a huge range of computer-based or tablet-based cognitive-training software programs or what most people call brain games. They promise you a sharper mind and a younger brain for longer. It must be my age, but I receive a *lot* of social media ads that tell me neurologists are *begging* people to play this or the other game. The ads sometimes prey on vulnerable people who are desperate to ward off or reverse dementia and any hint of an impending stint in a nursing home. They reassure us that their claims are based on solid 'scientific evidence' and are 'designed by neuroscientists' at top universities.

Do they work?

Well, yes. A bit. Different studies have yielded wildly differing results and even meta-analyses of the various trials have come to different conclusions.

I'm going to try to unpack this a bit for you now.

Some forms of cognitive training give you improvement in the specific skills being targeted in a given activity. And those benefits sometimes extend to improvements in other cognitive tasks administered by researchers. In some studies, the benefits for these specific skills are reported to stay around for years, while in others the benefits dwindle over time, often quite quickly once you stop doing the activities.

Making firm conclusions across the board on brain training as a whole is really difficult. One issue is that there is very little evidence that doing better on a set of cognitive tests in a study translates to delaying the onset of dementia in real life. Or that these skills help you remember to take your medication or remind you how to do your job so you can stay in the workforce.

Dr Loren Mowszowski is a clinical neuropsychologist who leads the Cognitive Training research stream within the specialised Healthy Brain Ageing Program at the University of Sydney's Brain and Mind Centre. She has led much research into cognitive training. She wonders whether it is the fact that we're not using the most appropriate tests in studies to evaluate the brain training programs that has led to us not getting the most out of them. 'So many tests we use are tests of new learning, not episodic memories,' she told me. 'Are we not quite seeing the benefits because the tests we're using are not quite getting it right?'

To illustrate her point, I am going to talk about a massive trial called the ACTIVE trial, which has spun off an entire suite of commercial brain-training activities based on the studies published from the trial data. But I think you will agree once you read this, the data is far from conclusive.

The ACTIVE trial has been going for over 10 years and is the most ambitious study so far to test different forms of cognitive training. The original goal of the study was to test whether different types of cognitive training could improve the daily life of older people in things like cooking and showering, as well as problem solving and cognitive performance.

Between March 1998 and October 1999, 2832 adults aged 65 years or older whose Mini-Mental State Examination (MMSE) scores were equal to or greater than a score of 23 (remember that's *not* dementia, although the test is deeply flawed), and who were still living at home, were enrolled in the trial. The participants were divided into three groups, with each group targeted to test a different skill. A control group of people who did not receive any cognitive training was also assigned for each group.

The cognitive training techniques were similar in that they all consisted of 10–14 sessions, each one lasting between 60 and 75 minutes over five to six weeks. The results *sound* super impressive. If you head to the ACTIVE study's website, you will see they have some pretty big claims. According to the study, '87 per cent of the participants who used BrainHQ's Double Decision [the commercial product the study has produced which targets speed of decisions] showed meaningful increases in the targeted cognitive ability, while 74 per cent of participants who used reasoning training and 26 per cent of those who used memory training showed improvements,' the site states. That sounds like a no-brainer. Sign me up now!

But not so fast! Independent researchers analysing the data have slightly different interpretations of the results. Certainly, the data at the 10-year mark showed the people who had received brain training reported that they were now doing better in their 'activities of daily living'. But on objective testing, their memory had not improved. Other areas that didn't really show improvements were processing speed, everyday problem-solving or reasoning.

And while the study participants who received any kind of training did a bit better after five years in the specific area they were trained in, that benefit didn't extend to other areas. For example, people who received reasoning and processing speed training (being able to do a mental task quickly) had fewer car accidents but didn't perform better in other areas. Importantly, over time, there was no difference in any group, including the control group, when it came to being diagnosed with dementia.

The ACTIVE trial has been criticised for being open to bias, as well as other issues. For example, after five years, 33 per cent of all the people in the trial had stopped participating and that number went up to 57 per cent after 10 years. To be fair, 18 per cent of the participants had passed away. Big dropout rates usually mean the data is skewed because if you're doing super well you tend to stay in the trial. The trial also didn't test for depression which can really skew the results.

So that's one big trial which has spawned a product. If you're buying a commercial brain-training program, you should be aware most apps available to consumers have not undergone scientific validation at all.

Maybe cognitive training is better when combined with physical exercise at the same time?

In 2021, a Swedish meta-analysis of 41 randomised trials of cognitive training for people both with and without mild cognitive impairment was published. In this meta-analysis 'simultaneous training' (which is where cognitive and physical training are done at the same time), was found to be the best approach for improving cognition, followed by 'sequential combinations' (cognitive then physical or vice versa) and then cognitive training alone. But the benefits were described as small.

I am trying to picture 14 sessions each lasting up to 75 minutes of cognitive training while on an exercise bike. It doesn't sound like much fun, or worth the effort for the small benefits on offer.

What the experts do to maintain brain health
DR LOREN MOWSZOWSKI

Loren is young and has two little children. She is focused on keeping her brain sharp. While her health is good, her family has a history of vascular disease. She gets her blood pressure, blood sugar and cholesterol levels checked through her GP yearly. She doesn't take any supplements but has a healthy diet. 'Exercise is something I'm not doing enough of,' she said. She also told me that while her drinking crept up during the pandemic, she's back to one glass of wine three nights a week. She is very proactive in protecting her mental health and her sleep.

Exergaming

Exergaming is defined as a combination of exercise and gaming. It's an innovative, fun and relatively safe way to exercise in a virtual reality or gaming environment. In 2020, a Chinese meta-analysis looked at 10 studies on the impact of exergaming on balance, gait, executive function and episodic memory for people with mild cognitive impairment and for dementia. The authors couldn't conclude they could see any benefits (which frankly is a relief – I know few people my age or older who enjoy gaming!).

So, are there easier and more pleasant ways to challenge our brains and still derive benefits?

Challenge your brain

Dr Loren Mowszowski says 'pushing your brain until it's uncomfortable' is good for neuroplasticity. She encourages all of us to exercise our brains as much as we can, not necessarily with a brain training app but more with simple activities that are different to what you usually do. 'You have to challenge your brain in different ways,' she advised and then confessed that as she was not a visual person, she had started doing arts and crafts with her children as a way of challenging the visual part of her brain.

Pick up a hobby ... or three!

Research done at Johns Hopkins University found that adults who regularly participated in a range of hobbies had between an 8 and 11 per cent reduction in the risk of memory impairment. In this study, reading books, magazines and newspapers, doing board games, crafts, crossword puzzles, jigsaw puzzles, playing musical instruments, bridge and other card games were all valid hobbies.

The Healthy Brain Project is a community-based initiative to understand optimal brain health and ageing. It is based out of the Turner Institute for Brain and Mental Health at Monash University. There are over 2000 Australians being followed up, with a focus on what makes a difference in midlife. And lots of researchers are dissecting the data that is coming out of this group. In February 2020, a new study from the Healthy Brain Project confirmed that doing a wide variety of cognitively stimulating leisure activities, is better for your cognitive performance than doing a smaller number of activities more often. In other words, variety matters more than frequency!

Dr Loren Mowszowski is a big fan of this kind of brain training. 'I advise my patients to pick up a new hobby. That might be something like backgammon.' She says so many of her patients know in theory that going to Italian classes or trying their hand at poetry would be a good thing to do for their brains but don't bother starting, fearing they will never become fluent in the language or good poets. But that's the wrong attitude. 'It is not about the mastery,' Loren insisted. 'It's about the experience! It's about the challenge!'

Dr Yen Ling Lim, the primary investigator of the Healthy Brain Project, agrees. 'Find something you're interested in and start with that,' she suggests. 'It almost doesn't matter what it is.'

What the experts do to maintain brain health
ASSOCIATE PROFESSOR YEN LING LIM

When I spoke to Yen she was into a deep love affair with Cross Fit. 'Lots of fitness regimes for women are geared towards weight loss and getting smaller. I've always had a very problematic relationship with my body image,' she said. She loves both the fact that there are no mirrors in a Cross Fit gym and the social value it brings. It's helped her sleep. She drinks neither coffee nor alcohol and has an all-round healthy diet. She doesn't take any supplements.

Social engagement

There is consistent scientific evidence that living alone and having no close relationships or having a very small social network have been linked to increased risk of dementia. But more importantly, the evidence shows that socialising is associated with reduced risk of dementia and increases in brain volume, even in adults with the APOE e4 gene (the most well studied gene that has been linked to a higher dementia risk). It turns out that socialising uses more neurons and neuronal connections than you'd think. So socialising is actually a brain workout. You have to concentrate on what the other people are saying, prepare your own thoughts and present them in a socially appropriate way while also reading other people's body language, facial expressions and tone.

Socialising doesn't need to be entertaining and/or involve going to parties. Just hanging out with friends, having a chat when you pick up some milk from the local shop, exercising in a group or participating in a book club is enough. As Professor Ian Hickie, of Sydney's Brain and Mind Centre, points out, staying in the (paid or unpaid) workforce usually has you mixing with your co-workers on a daily basis, stimulating your brain.

Socialising in midlife has immediate consequences. Studies done on people staying in Antarctica to study or a solo walker across the vast Australian Simpson Desert show that even short periods of isolation wreak havoc with your brain's cognition skills. A 13-week Scottish study done during the first COVID-19 lockdown in 2020 showed that it didn't take long for people to not only feel sadder but to display a decline in mental abilities. And the same study showed that the easing of restrictions led to an immediate benefit in terms of cognitive performance.

Stay in the workforce!

When I spoke to Professor Ian Hickie, he was emphatic about staying in the workforce in some capacity to delay the onset of MCI or dementia. Staying employed – even if you are not paid – is his number one hottest tip. While he is empathetic to people who are dreaming of a relaxed retirement that they imagine will look like an extended beach holiday, he is wary. '[For brain health], the worst thing in the world for active people in their 60s is to retire,' he says. 'If you think going to lie on a beach in Queensland is good for your health, you couldn't be more wrong.'

He says that being at work helps you use your brain. And it's not about the types of work you do. Even if you consider your job lowly paid, or boring, you are interacting with others, which is stimulating your brain. You are also following a routine, which we know also improves brain health indirectly through reinforcing and strengthening your circadian rhythms. (See Chapter 9 on sleep.)

All the over-60-year-old experts I spoke to for this book, including Dr Ian Hickie, Professor Victor Henderson of Stanford University, neurologist and author Dr David Perlmutter and Professor Dimity Pond of the University of Newcastle, work not just full-time but have a supersized workload. And they don't plan to exit stage left any time soon.

On the other hand, cognitive neurologist Dr Trevor Chong, from the Turner Institute for Brain and Mental Health at Monash University, doesn't see things that way. Having observed a number of colleagues and family members retire at age 65, only to get hit with a severe and sometimes ultimately fatal diagnosis, he is passionate about ensuring he retires in time to have meaningful time with his wife and children while he is healthy. Having said that, he plans to stay engaged in work in some capacity, even as a volunteer a couple of days a week to keep his brain healthy. He also cautions against staying in a job that requires significant cognitive agility beyond your use-by date. 'I'm going to tell my colleagues to tell me if they think something's not quite right,' he said.

Own a pet

As you get older, owning a pet, like a dog or cat, especially for five years or longer, was linked to slower cognitive decline, according to a study published in 2022. Perhaps it's the human–animal bond, which we know has health benefits like decreasing blood pressure and stress. It could be the fact that with some animals, you're forced to walk them, which increases your physical activity. Perhaps it's the fact that you have to get up each morning to feed them, keeping you set in a circadian rhythm.

For me, socialising, actively enjoying my work, gardening, bush-walking and hiking whenever I can are all amazing forms of keeping both my brain and body healthy. But I am not doing any brain-training games and nor were any of the brain experts I spoke to in researching this book.

Takeaways

- All the experts agreed that some form of regular exercise is beneficial for general health, which in turn is beneficial for your brain.
- Exercise doesn't have to mean the gym. It can include any form of movement you enjoy such as gardening, Tai Chi, bushwalking, dancing or even housework.
- Brain-training games are not necessarily the best way to keep your brain from declining. It all comes down to the act of challenging the brain on a regular basis, not how or what you use to do it.
- Social engagement and staying in the workforce for as long as possible have been proven to be beneficial to preventing MCI or dementia.
- Owning a pet has been linked to slower cognitive decline. So that's a yes to the new dog or cat (or even rabbit or bird)!

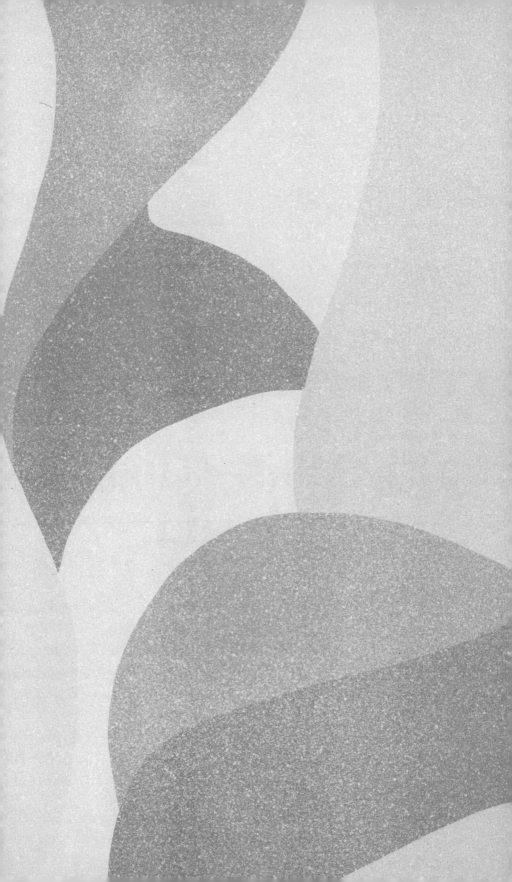

CHAPTER 5

What diet is best for protecting your brain?

They say you are what you eat and that holds true for your brain, too. For decades, people have been studying what the best diets and supplements are for preserving your brain. Despite this, a study published in 2022 found that, at least in the US, our diets are just getting worse year on year. It's a bit devastating.

A 2011 study showed that otherwise healthy university students who ate diets containing lots of fat and refined sugar performed worse on memory tasks that needed a properly functioning hippocampus. These same students were even less accurate at recalling what they had just eaten and were also less sensitive to hunger and satiety cues.

A diet higher in saturated fats and refined sugars, which is sometimes known as a 'Western diet' (we in 'the West' tend to have less fresh foods and more processed and junk foods), as opposed to the diets eaten in Asian, European or Middle-Eastern countries, has been specifically linked to a smaller left hippocampus in a 2015 study of 255 older adults.

What's going on here?

There are two pathways in which our diet impacts our brains. Eating healthy foods means our body can benefit from ingredients including antioxidants, vitamins, polyphenols and other nutrients. And some of these nutrients also have a critical role in brain function, immune system function and gene expression. You can think of your genes as recipes sitting in your DNA. Gene expression is the *process* where genes send out recipes to make RNA molecules. You've heard about RNA from all the COVID-19 vaccines, right? RNA acts as middlemen to decode the recipe and use it to make vital proteins (or sometimes does stuff itself). 'Gene expression' is like an 'on/off switch' to control when and where RNA molecules and their proteins are made. But they're also a bit of a 'volume control' to dial up and down the amount of protein made by a cell. Different conditions inside a cell determine gene expression and we are learning more about this all the time.

And here is the second – and possibly more interesting – pathway. Increasingly, the role of the bacterial bugs – and they can be both good and bad – in our guts (also known as our gut microbiota or sometimes the microbiome) is recognised as having a key role in the functioning of our physical and, subsequently, our mental health. Scientists now believe that a bad diet leads to a change in the microbiota, which then leads to inflammation – which is bad for our brains. Studies in rats and mice suggest that it's the hippocampus (the part of the brain responsible for memory) that's especially sensitive to inflammation.

We've known for a while that obesity itself, plus the diseases it is linked to such as type 2 diabetes mellitus and cardiovascular disease, are characterised by a state of chronic low-grade inflammation. Assessing a diet's 'inflammatory potential' is a fairly new concept. This is where foods are given a score for their pro- or anti-inflammatory effect on the body. That score is called the DII. Diets that are pro-inflammatory have a high DII score while anti-inflammatory diets have a low DII score. Diets with a high DII score are associated with higher risk of mild cognitive impairment (MCI) and generally poor cognitive outcomes.

But it's not *just* inflammation that is the problem. It is far more complex. We're now starting to piece together other chemical and physical links between a poor diet and the effects on the brain. Here's just one example: rodent and human diets high in fat and refined sugar have been found to reduce an important protein in our brains. This 'brain-derived neurotrophic factor (BDNF)' is a protein that helps protect and nurture synapses. Lower BDNF has been correlated with memory deficits.

Studies have confirmed that your gut microbiota is the key that links poor diet and low levels of BDNF. It does this by altering the amount and types of key short chain fatty acids (SCFAs) in the gut and therefore the brain. Scientists are *right now* studying how we might be able to use probiotics and prebiotics to help our brains out.

What about your weight?

Before we delve into the specifics of different diets, I'm going to put in a word for just staying in your healthy weight range. Studies have shown that in middle age, obesity is linked with subsequent cognitive impairment and that's independent of any other health-related factors. Why? Well, obesity raises your risk for a number of medical problems, like metabolic syndrome, general inflammation and cardiovascular disease. These in turn increase your risk of dementia. Remember that if it's good for the heart, it's good for the brain, and vice versa. But it might be that the same lack of exercise and bad diet that causes obesity also causes dementia. Regardless, if you have a healthy body weight, you're less likely to develop cognitive issues.

Specific diets for a healthy brain

So which diet should you be on to preserve your brain? We are going to look at ketogenic diets, diets known as 'anti-inflammatory' diets including the Mediterranean diet, the DASH diet (which began as a diet specifically targeting high blood pressure) and the MIND diet (a combination of the Mediterranean and the DASH diet), as well as plant-based and vegetarian diets. We will also touch on caloric restriction.

The ketogenic diet

A ketogenic (or 'keto') diet is a low-carbohydrate, high-fat diet. In fact, fats make up around 90 per cent of the calories on this diet. This means that the body is forced to burn fat as its main source of fuel. It then breaks this fat down into 'ketone bodies' or 'ketones', in a process called ketosis. Keto diets are super effective as a weight-loss strategy (people lose on average up to 5 per cent of body weight in six months). We don't know exactly why it's so effective, but there's some evidence that because you are fuller for longer from eating such a high percentage of fats, you tend to eat far fewer calories overall.

What does a keto diet do for the brain? According to neurologist and author Dr David Perlmutter, ketones act as an important source of energy for the brain. 'The primary fuel of the brain is glucose [carbohydrate or sugar],' he explained. But the ability to use ketones in the brain for fuel derives from our ancestors, who were at constant risk of starvation. 'With starvation, your body's metabolism begins to shift quite aggressively,' Dr Perlmutter says. Because your brain cells can't use fats for metabolism, when the brain runs out of glucose, it switches to the back-up nutrients – ketones. Ketones can be really exceptional for fuelling the brain, and Dr Perlmutter pointed me to a study that showed more mitochondria development in the hippocampus of rats on a keto diet.

Ketones are available to the brain not only when glucose is in short supply but also when the brain's metabolism is faulty (as it is in Alzheimer's disease). Back in the 1920s, neurologists noticed that epileptic patients had way fewer seizures after a period of fasting. There are now a few – albeit small – studies showing that strictly sticking to a keto diet can help reduce your dementia risk.

On a keto diet you would eat as few wholegrains and legumes as possible, in stark contrast with the Mediterranean diet (see page 98). Also off the menu are wine and beer. That counts me out. But if you are a carnivore, this diet may be for you. It encourages lots of meat, including the red meat shunned by most of the other healthy brain diets.

Dr Joanna McMillan is a PhD qualified nutrition scientist. She's also an Adjunct Senior Research Fellow with La Trobe University and a guest lecturer at the University of Sydney. Keto is not her diet of choice, but she doesn't dismiss it. However, she says that if you're going to do the keto diet, you have to commit. 'I get people telling me, "I do keto one day a week." But you're not going to hit ketosis in one day,' she explained. 'It takes a week!' That's because your body still has plentiful supplies of glycogen — a long-term storage form of sugar found in muscles and the liver — to go through before it needs to tuck into your fat stores and make ketones.

What the experts do to maintain brain health
DR DAVID PERLMUTTER

David drinks a glass of red wine every two to three days and eats mainly oily fish and rarely red meat or dairy. He monitors his sleep on an Oura ring and takes a daily evening walk with his wife. He also uses supplements including nicotinamide riboside, sulforaphane plus myrosinase, turmeric plus black pepper, a multivitamin, vitamin D, a probiotic and prebiotic and epicatechin.

KETOGENIC DIETS HAVE SOME MAJOR DOWNSIDES
They're high in saturated fat. And diets high in saturated fats have been linked in several studies to heart disease, as well as higher levels of 'bad' LDL cholesterol, which is also linked to heart disease and strokes. No point dying early of a heart attack with an intact brain, right!?

They're also linked to deficiencies of some nutrients. Because you eat close to no carbohydrates, you often have very few fruits and vegetables on a keto diet. Dieticians warn this could lead to deficiencies in some important micronutrients, such as vitamins B and C, magnesium, phosphorus and selenium.

Then there's the famous 'keto flu'. As your body begins its transition period of switching over from glucose for fuel to ketones, it can make you feel like you are getting something like the flu. The symptoms include light-headedness, fatigue, headaches, and nausea. As carbohydrates are restricted and glycogen stores are depleted, the body rapidly depletes its stores of sodium and fluids. Increasing sodium by 1–2 g per day may help.

Last but not least, I have to mention the constipation. The keto diet can be low in fibre because of the low vegetable, grain and legumes intake. There are a lucky few who can poop for the nation even on a keto diet low in fibre. That's awesome. For the rest of us, I think there are easier diets around with better evidence to support their impact on brain health.

The Mediterranean diet

The Mediterranean diet was first defined by Ancel Keys, an American doctor who specialised in studying the impacts of diet on health in the 1960s. His Mediterranean diet is based on the eating habits of the people in Greece and Southern Italy. As a rule, people who stick to this diet have a high intake of extra virgin olive oil, vegetables including leafy green vegetables, fruits, cereals, nuts, pulses or legumes, moderate amounts of fish and other meat, dairy products and red wine, and low intake of eggs and sweets. This type of diet has been found to be anti-inflammatory.

As you know well by now, inflammation has been strongly implicated as a major cause of dementia. So, reducing inflammation in the brain and body has been a major target of researchers. Of all the experts and brain gurus I spoke to, the most common diet pattern followed is the Mediterranean diet.

The diet has been specifically studied as an intervention to ward off dementia and it looks good. A US study of 121 people reported that those who stuck to the Mediterranean diet had better learning and memory and better-looking MRI scans. One 2018 study of 116 older New Yorkers found that those who stuck to a Mediterranean diet had a much thicker cerebral cortex than those on a typical Western diet.

> ### What the experts do to maintain brain health
> ### DR JOANNA MCMILLAN
>
> Joanna follows a Mediterranean diet but augments that with krill oil supplements (even though she does eat oily fish), as well as Tru Niagen, 300 mg once a day. This supplement contains nicotinamide riboside chloride and is designed to increase your levels of NAD+. She is quite the exerciser, going to the gym and walking with friends most days. 'Walking is my meditation,' she told me.
>
> 'My one vice is my wine,' she admitted. A red wine, especially a pinot noir, is often a nightly ritual. But she stops at one to two glasses. She then switches to tea. Coffee? A firm yes – up till 2 pm. For the sake of her sleep that's the end of caffeine for the day for Joanna.

And in 2013, a meta-analysis of 12 studies found the diet is linked to slower cognitive decline and a lower risk of developing Alzheimer's disease.

Given that this type of diet also reduces your risk of cancer, heart disease and diabetes and improves your chances of living just a longer life in general, it's hard to argue against it!

The DASH (Dietary Approaches to Stop Hypertension) diet

The DASH diet doesn't include specific foods but rather has a few basic principles. They include eating vegetables, fruit and wholegrains, as well as incorporating fat-free or low-fat dairy products, fish, poultry, beans, nuts and vegetable oils. It also suggests limiting foods that are high in saturated fat, such as fatty meats, full-fat dairy products and tropical oils like coconut, palm kernel and palm oils, as well as sugar-sweetened drinks and sweets. Sounds simple enough.

Studies show that the DASH diet can lower your blood pressure within two to four weeks, after which it tends to keep you at this lower level, rather than continue to lower your blood pressure further. This diet can also reduce your risk of cardiovascular disease by 13 per cent and reduce the rate of diabetes and obesity. Studies also show that people who follow a DASH-type diet have less MCI and dementia over time. Other studies show that switching someone with cognitive decline to a DASH diet reduces their rate of further cognitive decline.

But could there be an even better diet? Maybe!

The MIND (Mediterranean-DASH Intervention for Neurodegenerative Delay) diet

The MIND diet was developed with the specific aim of keeping the brain younger. It was developed by Dr Martha Clare Morris, a nutritional epidemiologist from Rush University, Chicago.

Like the DASH diet, the MIND diet isn't prescriptive on exactly what to eat but rather incorporates 10 healthy-brain food groups, which are listed on the next page:

What diet is best for protecting your brain?

1. **Green leafy vegetables.** This is somewhat unique to the MIND diet, in that green leafy veggies like kale, spinach and lettuce are singled out in lowering the risk of dementia and cognitive decline. This is probably not surprising given that green vegetables like broccoli, beans or spinach are packed with nutrients linked to better brain health, such as folate, vitamin E, carotenoids and flavonoids. On the MIND diet, aim to eat *at least six servings of leafy greens a week.*
2. **Other vegetables:** aim for at least one serve a day (FYI a serve is half a cup of cooked or one cup of raw vegetables).
3. **Nuts:** aim for five servings a week (i.e. one serve is 30 g).
4. **Berries:** aim for at least two servings a week.
5. **Beans:** aim for at least three servings a week.
6. **Wholegrains:** aim for at least three servings a day (i.e. half a cup of cooked rice or pasta, 1 slice of bread).
7. **Fish:** aim for once a week.
8. **Poultry:** aim for twice a week.
9. **Olive oil.** The amount isn't specified but the idea is that you use it as your main cooking oil.
10. **Wine.** Although the type of wine is not specified, most experts believe that red wine has more antioxidants than white, possibly because of contact of the wine with the nutrient-loaded grape skins. On this diet you get a glass a day!

It also identifies five unhealthy food groups to avoid:

1. Red meats.
2. Butter and margarine.
3. Cheese.
4. Pastries and sweets.
5. Fried/fast food.

Here is a comparison of the three diets that have been studied according to their impact on brain health, so their differences and similarities can be easily identified.

DASH	MEDITERRANEAN	MIND
Total grains at least 7 serves per day	Non-refined grains at least 4 or more serves per day	Wholegrains 3 or more serves per day
Vegetables at least 4 or more serves per day	Vegetables ≥ 4 serves per day, potatoes > 2 serves per day	Green leafy vegetables ≥ 6 serves per week, other vegetables ≥ 2 serves per day
Fruits ≥ 4 serves per day	Fruits ≥ 3 serves per day	Berries ≥ 2 serves per week
Dairy ≥ 2 serves per day	Full fat dairy ≤ 10 serves per week	Cheese < 1 serve per week; butter, margarine < 1 tbs per day
Meat, poultry & fish ≤ 2 serves per day	Red meat ≤ 1 serve per week, fish > 6 serves per week, poultry ≤ 3 serves per week	Red meat & red meat products < 4 serves per week, fish ≥ 1 serve per week, poultry ≥ 2 serves per week
Nuts, seeds & legumes ≥ 4 serves per week	Legumes, nuts and beans > 6 serves per week	Beans > 3 serves per week, nuts ≥ 5 serves per week
Total fat ≤ 27% of kcal, saturated fat ≤ 6% of kcal	Olive oil ≥ 1 serve per day	Olive oil is the primary oil
No guidelines for wine	Wine 1–2 glasses per day	Wine 1 glass per day

These diets haven't been compared directly to each other in a study. In other words, nobody has taken three very similar groups of people, put one group on the DASH diet, one on the MIND diet one on the Mediterranean diet, followed them up and compared their rates of dementia. Each diet is done in a silo. So it's really hard to be certain which diet steps up as the gold star winner!

Plant-based diets

In 2018, the controversial documentary *The Game Changers* hit Netflix and it felt like everyone was talking about eating a plant-based diet. Daniel and I also decided to adopt this way of eating. I can't say it was just because of the documentary – which used very dubious science – but mainly we realised that we had been eating fewer vegetables than we should and because the carbon footprint of eating meat made us feel guilty. Plus, many of the diets that have reportedly good health benefits, such as the Mediterranean, MIND and DASH diets, could all nearly be described as largely plant-based. For me, there wasn't a huge change to my diet other than upping the veggie content. It meant having a salad with some egg, fish or tofu rather than just pasta with a vegetarian sauce. For Daniel, it was a *huge* turnaround. The guy loves a BBQ. Or did.

I remember doing an Instagram post on this and receiving lots of push back from people saying plant-based eating is just a vegan diet. In fact, it's not been terribly well defined. The Australian Heart Foundation describes plant-based eating as including 'a range of eating patterns from eating no animal products to including small-to-moderate amounts of animal products'.

The lack of proper definition has made it hard to find good research data to support this way of eating in order to protect your brain health.

In one group of 6525 people aged between 65 and 110 years and already enrolled in the Chinese Longitudinal Healthy Longevity Survey, the authors found that living in polluted areas was associated with a 46 per cent increase in the risk of developing poor cognitive function. However, eating a plant-based diet was the thing that protected these people from the effects of pollution on their brains.

At this stage it appears the jury is still out on the benefits of eating a plant-based diet. But it seems to me that the DASH, Mediterranean and MIND diets could all easily be plant-based.

Caloric restriction (AKA just eating less!)

Placing mice and rats on a tight calorie-restricted diet has proven to be great for their little rodent brains. In humans, especially the more portly among us, strict calorie-restricted diets have been found to effectively contribute to weight loss, and improve general health, sleep quality and sexual function for people needing to lose a certain amount of weight. But the evidence of calorie restriction for improving brain health is sketchy. Possibly because maintaining caloric restriction long term is just so tough!

While there were improvements in cognitive functions, such as verbal recognition and memory, as shown in a study conducted over a two-year period, and there was a decline in the production of BDNF, the results could not determine if the effects were sustainable past this time. The main limiting factor seems to be the ability for subjects to restrict their calories long-term (something most of us know about already!).

A high-fibre diet

Back in the 1980s, a group of Japanese researchers started following a group of almost 4000 people aged between 40 and 60 years. The research group released its latest findings in 2022. At the outset of the study, the researchers asked the study participants to report on their last 24 hours of eating. Over the 20 odd years of the study, about 670 of these people got dementia. I was struck by the finding that the people who ate the least amount of fibre also had a higher development rate of dementia. This was especially true of soluble fibre.

Let me explain what that means. Fibre is all the parts of plant foods your body can't digest or absorb. So, it just keeps travelling through the gut to the large bowel. Soluble fibre dissolves in water, forming a gel-like substance. It helps lower cholesterol and glucose levels. You find soluble fibre in oats, peas, beans like black beans, Brussels sprouts, apples, carrots and barley. Insoluble fibre doesn't dissolve in water and travels intact through the guts. It acts as a bulking agent, giving you a nice big stool. Nuts, wholegrains and vegetables like cauliflower, as well as pulses and lentils, green beans and potatoes, are all good examples.

The researchers pointed out that the higher the participants' fibre intake, especially the soluble type, the lower the body weight, the systolic blood pressure, cholesterol and glucose levels. The risk of stroke and diabetes was also lower. All of this would indirectly help prevent dementia. The researchers also pointed out that a Mediterranean diet is high in fibre, and that high-fibre diets often naturally combine with good fats and a high level of nutrients. 'One possibility is that soluble fibre regulates the composition of gut bacteria. This composition may affect neuroinflammation, which plays a role in the onset of dementia,' the lead author, Kazumasa Yamagishi of the University of Tsukuba, suggested in a release that went with the study.

My diet advice

As there is not one diet that seems to be an outright winner in protecting your brain against developing MCI or dementia, I suggest you pick a style of eating that suits you and offers the best benefits for your overall health. You can also pick and choose from the different diets. For example, I have cherrypicked the MIND diet's foods to avoid and basically don't include four of them in my diet. But cheese is non-negotiable for me. Armed with the DASH and Mediterranean diet advice, I am still eating cheese and enjoying it. In doing so I'm also ensuring I have adequate calcium for my bones. I have gone with the DASH diet's four plus serves of veggies a day. (I admit I just can't do six serves of leafy greens!) I'm drinking wine every night (just one glass) and feeling pious about it instead of guilty. All the oil we use is olive oil.

Drink enough water

There is some evidence that people who are always a bit dehydrated damage their arteries and develop high blood pressure. Being dehydrated also directly impairs your brain function, as well as your ability to exert yourself when exercising.

But how much water do you actually need? Women need to drink 2.1 litres of fluid a day, in addition to any food consumed; men need 2.6 litres. You will need more if you are sweating a lot or if you are pregnant or breastfeeding.

Takeaways

- While there is no one proven diet that protects against dementia, the anti-inflammatory diets such as the Mediterranean, MIND and DASH diets all appear to offer evidence in slowing the progress of MCI and Alzheimer's.
- Plant-based diets don't just mean vegetarian or vegan diets. The Mediterranean, MIND and DASH diets could all be modified to be plant-based.
- A diet that is good for our heart is also good for our brain health.
- Women need 2.1 litres of water a day while men need 2.6.

CHAPTER 6

Brain health in a pill?

A word of warning: while I don't take any supplements myself and wouldn't recommend them, that is not a universal view and they are very popular. While I examine a range of supplements and drinks in this section, the only ones that I actually take are wine, tea and coffee. So, if you want to dive into the weeds a little about some of the more common brain supplements and the current (mostly lack of) evidence around them – read on. If not, you can take a short cut to the next chapter.

I've always been an advocate for getting your vitamins from your food. But I didn't want my biases to taint my ideas about the potential role of supplements for brain health. So I turned to the experts.

Victor Henderson is Professor of Epidemiology and Population Health and of Neurology and Neurological Sciences at Stanford University in California. His research focuses on risk factors for cognitive ageing and neurodegenerative dementia, and on interventions to help prevent and treat these disorders. He also directs the Stanford Alzheimer's Disease Research Center, principally funded by the National Institute of Health (NIH). *Spoiler alert*: he doesn't take any supplements. *None*. 'There are so many things that make good sense scientifically. For example, they may reduce inflammation. But whether or not they have any clinical effects is another thing entirely,' he told me. 'I'm really sceptical about all of them.' He says so many supplements make promises they simply cannot prove. 'If they really believe they work, go to the NIH for funding and do the research!' He says patients constantly ask him for recommendations around supplements. He can't give them any.

On the other hand we have Professor David Sinclair, a famous anti-ageing specialist based at Harvard University, where he is co-director of the Paul F. Glenn Center for Biology of Aging Research. He's gone on the record with the list of supplements he takes daily (which must be noted is for longevity and not specifically brain health). These are based on much of his own research. Let's take a look at what's on Professor Sinclair's supplement list.

- 1 g NMN (nicotinamide mononucleotide)
- 1 g resveratrol every morning with caffeinated coffee
- 250 mg quercetin
- vitamins D + K2
- 1 g Metformin at night
- high-dose statin (for his genetically driven high cholesterol).

NMN (nicotinamide mononucleotide) or (NR) nicotinamide riboside

About a year ago, my neighbour dropped off a leaflet about the NMN supplement she was taking. I'd never heard of it. Then my friend and colleague Dr Joanna McMillan told me that she takes it for brain health, just like Professor Sinclair.

I was intrigued! I immediately started looking into the science behind this supplement. Here are my findings. (Bear with me – this is one for the science nerds.)

Nicotinamide adenine dinucleotide (aka NAD+) is a coenzyme essential for energy metabolism in the cell. Levels of NAD+ availability decrease with age. And there is increasing evidence showing that this plays a massive role in cell ageing. Still with me? Studies show that a lack of NAD+ is also linked to a whole raft of chronic diseases from type 2 diabetes to obesity, heart failure to Alzheimer's disease.

Nicotinamide riboside (NR) and nicotinamide mononucleotide (NMN) are both used by your body to make NAD+. The theory is that if you supplement with NMN or NR you could boost your NAD and get healthier cells. NMN must be converted to NR to get into the cell, so it makes sense to talk about NR and NMN together.

There are a ton of studies that show various benefits of NMN or NR supplements on a variety of rodents. Wistar rats (albino rats commonly used in laboratory tests) seem to fare especially well. Human trials? Apparently, they're coming but they're not here yet. That hasn't stopped a lot of companies going out to market with NMN and NR products and making all sorts of claims that are frankly well ahead of the science. We don't know whether either does anything in humans yet, and apart from that, we don't even know how much to take, when, for how long or for which conditions.

You can actually get NMN from your diet. It is naturally found in cabbage, cucumber, broccoli, tomato, mushrooms and avocado. So my advice is to add these NMN-rich veggies into your brain-healthy diet we've just discussed in the previous chapter. Forget the supplements and save your money.

Quercetin

Found naturally in tomatoes, apples and tea, quercetin is a flavonoid or a powerful antioxidant. Tests conducted in a Petri dish show that it seems to protect neurons from oxidative damage while reducing lipid peroxidation (the breakdown of the cell membrane causing inevitable cell destruction). It is thought to help with athletic performance, heart and blood vessel diseases, arthritis and diabetes, among other things. It also seems to prevent the formation of amyloid-β proteins and prevent inflammation in the cell. While there are many studies that measure its impact on parts of the process important in maintaining (or losing) brain health, they all describe how it *could* help ward off brain disease, but not whether it *actually does so*.

In addition to this, a large US study published in 2020 looking at diets rich in quercetins found that people consuming them naturally (i.e. via food) didn't reduce their risk of dementia.

My conclusion? Don't bother!

Resveratrol

Resveratrol is a polyphenol (also an antioxidant) found in grape skins and in dark red wines, as well as in peanuts, soy and berries.

Studies using cell cultures or animals do indeed show that resveratrol helps reduce oxidative stress and inflammation, suppressing overgrowth of the muscles that line blood vessels and contribute to high blood pressure. Resveratrol also promotes autophagy, which is the body's way of cleaning out damaged cells in order to regenerate newer, healthier ones. In human clinical trials, resveratrol reduced systolic blood pressure (that's the top number) in people with a higher blood pressure – a *little* bit. It has also reduced blood glucose in patients with diabetes.

The effects of resveratrol on the brain have been studied but only in animal and pre-clinical studies so far. Much of the focus has been around its ability to activate sirtuins, which are proteins found in human cells as well as plant cells, and also in soy beans, cocoa beans and some spices. Sirtuins help not only with controlling metabolism but also cell survival and repair, and extending the lifespan of a cell. They are like monitors checking each cell's viability and regulating the activity of key metabolic enzymes, as well as the activity of many genes. Resveratrol supplements were found to activate SIRT 1 and increased the lifespan and improved the health of several species of mice. In a Petri dish, human fibroblast cells exposed to resveratrol were slower to die off.

But can you conclude from this that it's a supplement worth taking? Put your wallet away – for now. There are human studies that do establish a link between consumption of foods rich in resveratrol (such as the red wine found in the Mediterranean and MIND diets) and lower odds of getting dementia, as well as improvements in learning, memory, visual and spatial orientation, and social skills. *But* it's hard to put that down to resveratrol alone, rather than the entire Mediterranean diet, and even if we did, that would be evidence for the food, not the supplement.

There have been a few studies done in humans and they're a mixed bag in terms of results. A six-month study in 56 people found that 200 mg of resveratrol a day showed greater improvement of verbal memory in healthy older adults than in those taking a placebo. On the other hand, a study in 60 young adults didn't show any meaningful cognitive benefits from taking 500 mg a day of resveratrol supplements for a month. In 2020, a placebo-controlled trial of 129 post-menopausal women that took resveratrol at a dose of 75 mg twice a day for 12 months showed that they had better blood flow to their brains and more improvements in their cognition than the women taking a placebo.

In none of the trials have we seen many negative side effects from resveratrol. But it is expensive. I had me a spot of online shopping and found all sorts of doses and all sorts of package sizes for all sorts of prices. While it looks promising, we don't know what dose should be taken, for how long or when, and we also must take into account that the studies done so far are tiny. I'd hold your horses till we have more proof.

Vitamin K2

Vitamin K is also known as phylloquinone, and it is found in green leafy vegetables like kale and spinach. Vitamin K2 (known as menaquinone) is also a natural form of vitamin K, and is found in meat, eggs and cheese as well as fermented vegetables (where it is synthesised by bacteria).

Two studies of the effects of anaesthetics on the brains of mice with dementia found that vitamin K2 raised ATP levels (the cell's way of storing energy) and helped prevent some of the cognitive impairment that usually results from anaesthesia. Staying with the rodents, low consumption of vitamin K1 in the diet resulted in cognitive deficits in rats in a small study. There is a bit of human data as well. One Irish study found that among a group of elderly people, the lowest consumption of vitamin K and the lowest blood levels of vitamin K were linked to a lower level of cognition. Mind you, the researchers were also monitoring inflammation, which was correlated with cognitive impairment, too. As they were studied together it's hard to know what to make of that. And just to confuse things a little more, in a study of 599 participants aged between 55 and 65, lower blood vitamin K levels was associated with a higher score for information processing speed . . . yes, *higher*! I'd say that at this stage the jury is out.

Now let's look at some other supplements you might see out there (not taken by Professor Sinclair).

Omega-3 fatty acids (omega-3s)

There are lots of good reasons to suggest that omega-3s are essential for the brain. For a start, some (but certainly not all) observational studies show that diets high in omega-3s lower the risk of mild cognitive impairment, Alzheimer's disease and other forms of dementia. Omega-3s form vital components of cell membranes. They are also especially in demand by the brain, the retina (back of the eye), and sperm. Your body uses omega-3s to make key signalling molecules which are critical for nerve function including inducing sleep and spatial learning, as well as having anti-inflammatory and neuroprotective properties.

The Mediterranean diet is packed with oily fish (a source of omega-3s). And many studies have shown that adding long chain omega-3s to baby formula (think Gold formulas) improves cognition in babies.

So there are reasons to believe that having some oily fish and plant-based sources of omega-3 in your diet makes sense . . . but what about when they come in the form of supplements?

Omega-3 supplements

Among the many scientists who have studied whether omega-3 supplements protect your brain is Dr Hussein Yassine, Associate

Professor in the Department of Medicine, Keck School of Medicine at the University of Southern California. He points to the powerful anti-inflammatory properties of omega-3 fats.

However, studies of fish oil and omega-3 as supplements for cognitive health have been disappointing, Dr Yassine says. Results from clinical trials have shown that omega-3 supplements don't really do anything to preserve cognitive function in older adults who start taking them when their brains are still functioning well. While there have been some positive results seen in people with mild MCI, there has been nothing of any significance seen in people with Alzheimer's. In addition, the studies and trials conducted so far have been small in size, poor quality and differ in the supplement regimes used. It is hard to conclude there is any real benefit yet.

Omega-3 vs omega-6 fatty acids

This is still a bit controversial, but Dr Yassine says apart from just increasing the amount of omega-3s in your diet, you might want to consider having a positive balance of omega-3s relative to the other polyunsaturated fatty acid, omega-6. But not all forms of omega-6 are friendly towards the brain. Eicosadienoic acid (a form of omega-6) actually tends to contribute to inflammation, cause constriction of blood vessels, and disrupts the action of platelets (blood clotting factor), which can cause blood clots to form. Avoiding them isn't easy. They're found in many nutritious foods like nuts, seeds and vegetable oils. This has been behind the push to use mainly olive oil instead of canola or blended vegetable oils.

So, bottom line . . . should you take a fish oil supplement?

'The supportive evidence isn't very strong,' says Dr Yassine. On the whole, trying to pick individual nutrients from a healthy food is fraught. 'If you isolate one active you won't get the same bang for your buck.' Sure, oily fish has lots of omega-3s. 'But they also have vitamins B and E, as well as lutein,' he says. He also says that people who eat a lot of salmon often have a healthier lifestyle too, which creates a synergistic effect. 'Trying to reduce brain health to a single food is too reductionist,' he insists.

In case you were wondering, the guru of omega-3 research for brain health *doesn't* take supplements. In fact, he takes no supplements at all, going instead for a healthy diet. 'I eat fatty fish once a week,' he told me. For people who can't stomach oily fish, supplements might be worth considering but Dr Yassine warns we have no evidence to say how much and how often to take them.

> What the experts do to maintain brain health
> ## ASSOCIATE PROFESSOR HUSSEIN YASSINE
>
> Hussein exercises two to three times a week for 30 minutes at a time. He tries to eat a well-rounded balanced diet and includes fatty fish once a week, plus pecans, walnuts and almonds for his omega-3s. He doesn't take any supplementary vitamins and drinks coffee and alcohol.

Curcumin

Curcumin, the active ingredient in turmeric, is a powerful antioxidant. It also has been shown to have anti-inflammatory and neuroprotective effects in the body. Studies in rats and in Petri dishes are promising but we don't have any real evidence that taking a curcumin supplement will help protect the brain from cognitive decline or depression.

B vitamins (folic acid and B12)

Folic acid is the natural form of vitamin B9. It is essential for your cells to form DNA and RNA (your unique genetic recipe codes stored in every single cell) as well as protein metabolism. It plays a key role in breaking down homocysteine, an amino acid that can have harmful effects in the body if its level rises too high. High homocysteine levels have been linked to a higher risk of arterial disease and strokes, but also specifically dementia and Alzheimer's disease. You get folic acid naturally from fruits and veggies, especially dark green leafy vegetables (think spinach and kale). It's also added into a lot of foods like bread and breakfast cereals.

Vitamin B12 is required for the development, myelination (process of forming a myelin or insulation sheath around a nerve to allow it to process messages more quickly) and function of the central nervous system, as well as healthy red blood cell formation and DNA synthesis. You get it naturally from animal products – think meat, chicken, seafood, eggs and dairy. Vitamin B12 deficiency produces an anaemia identical to that of folic acid deficiency but also causes irreversible damage to the brain and peripheral nervous systems. Symptoms can include burning or tingling in the feet from damaged nerves.

These two vitamins are often combined in supplements targeted at brain health. However, this was studied by a 2008 Cochrane review. Cochrane reviews are considered the pinnacle of medical research when experts come together to pick apart all the published studies and make a recommendation based on the evidence. The authors of this Cochrane review concluded that there was 'no evidence that folic acid with or without vitamin B12 improves cognitive function' in random elderly people with or without dementia. They did go on to say that 'long-term supplementation may benefit cognitive function of healthy older people with high homocysteine levels'. Vitamin B12, Vitamin B6 and folic acid helps breaks down homocysteine into useful chemicals used by the body. When things are working properly, there should be very low levels of homocysteine left in the blood. If you have high levels of homocysteine, you could have a deficiency in one of these vitamins, and it can also be a sign of heart disease, or a rare inherited disorder.

You can get a homocysteine blood test as part of a routine blood test from your GP. And given that vegans and some vegetarians have diets very low in B12, it is at least worth having a blood test to see where your levels are at and taking a supplement if needed. It's rarer but I do sometimes see people with folic acid deficiencies. You really need a horrible diet with very few veggies for this to happen, but if that's you, a simple blood test will pick that up, too.

Multivitamins

In 2018, a Cochrane review on vitamin and mineral supplementation was published that comprised data from 28 studies with more than 83,000 participants. The experts' conclusion? 'We did not find evidence that any vitamin or mineral supplementation strategy for cognitively healthy adults in mid or late life has a meaningful effect on cognitive decline or dementia, although the evidence does not permit definitive conclusions.' But before we get too dismissive, the review did point out that there wasn't conclusive data about people starting a supplement before the age of 60. Plus, the studies were usually too short to generate good data on long-term outcomes for cognitive function.

The massive COSMOS trial (COcoa Supplement and Multivitamin Outcomes Study) is an ongoing randomised clinical trial of 22,000 people that is looking at a cocoa extract supplement (containing a total of 500 mg/d flavanols, including 80 mg epicatechins), and a multivitamin supplement to reduce the risk of cardiovascular disease in older people. The average age at entry into this study was 73. A spin-off study (COSMOS-Mind) is looking at whether the cocoa extract supplement or the multivitamin supplement improves cognitive function and reduces the risk of cognitive impairment and dementia.

The team presented their initial findings in November 2021. It was found that the older participants who took a daily multivitamin had higher cognitive test scores after three years than those participants who took a placebo. (It wasn't such good news for the cocoa trial, unfortunately.) The results for the multivitamin were seriously impressive. The investigators estimated that multivitamins were slowing cognitive ageing by 60 per cent over the three years of the trial so far, reducing brain age by 1.8 years. The trial participants with a history of pre-existing cardiovascular disease at the start seemed to benefit most from the multivitamins.

The theory was that a lot of older adults often ate poorly and ended up with nutrient deficiencies, especially in B12, folate, vitamin D, and other micronutrients that have been linked to accelerated cognitive decline and dementia in other observational studies.

Multivitamins are cheap and well tolerated. It is not a bad idea to take one in older age as the impetus to shop for and cook healthy meals starts to slide.

Iron

As well as being vital to transporting oxygen around the body, iron also has a key role as the central molecule in the haem component of haemoglobin. It is critical for a metabolic process called oxidative phosphorylation. This is when cells use enzymes to oxidise nutrients that then release chemical energy to perform various biological functions. Plus, it is required for the production of myelin (the insulation sheaths around each nerve), and both the production and breakdown of neurotransmitters.

Lots of women are familiar with iron because we tend to lose it once a month during our periods until we hit menopause. Low iron is a common problem for premenopausal women. But the story changes as you get older. As you age, blood tests become less reliable: although we see your iron levels in your blood gradually decrease, your body's iron stores actually increase! That's because the systems that harvest and store iron when you're young don't switch off and, instead of efficiently shedding any excess iron (through having a period), it is stored and can accumulate in tissues, including your brain.

Professor Ashley Bush is the Director of the Melbourne Dementia Research Centre and Head of the Oxidation Biology Unit. He has done an enormous amount of research on metals and the brain, and has a specific interest in iron and its metabolism. 'We need iron supplies to be abundant in development because we have to synthesise so much haem, which is needed for the growth of the brain,' he explained. But the accumulation of iron in the brain as we age directly correlates with cognitive decline. The more iron in the brain, the greater that decline. '[The levels of] CSF ferritin is a very good predictor of cognitive decline,' Professor Bush says.

What the experts do to maintain brain health
PROFESSOR ASHLEY BUSH

Ashley exercises vigorously five days a week. Since his mid-40s he takes multiple supplements including vitamin E, selenium, C-Q10, fish oil and N-acetyl-cysteine to increase his glutathione levels. He drinks coffee and alcohol.

Before you panic and start throwing away the iron supplements you're taking for low iron, relax! 'The blood–brain barrier is very efficient at shutting out excess iron from accumulating in the brain,' says Professor Bush. But if those systems fail over a prolonged period of time, you might be in trouble.

Bottom line: if your doctor has diagnosed you with iron deficiency from a blood test and has advised you to take a short course of an iron supplement, you won't accidentally be giving yourself dementia.

Zinc

Zinc acts as a coenzyme for multiple enzymes involved with growth, immune function, cognitive function and bone function. Zinc has actually been shown to alter the β-amyloid plaques by changing the β-amyloid proteins into a form that is less harmful to the brain, especially in people with the APOE e4 gene. If you remember back to Chapter 2, we talked about the APOE gene making a protein that helps the brain's microglia clear excessive β-amyloid from the brain. Well, it seems that lower zinc levels inside brain cells might be partially responsible if this process becomes dysfunctional.

Studies have shown that people with Alzheimer's disease are more likely than people without to have zinc deficiency in both the blood and the cerebrospinal fluid (or CSF).

Getting zinc from your diet can be a bit tough if you don't like oysters, red meat or poultry. Some studies have found that one in three elderly people are zinc deficient. This might lead you to think that a zinc supplement would be a good idea. Maybe. Studies of zinc supplementation as a treatment for Alzheimer's disease in mice found they led to less β-amyloid and tau accumulation in the brain and less measurable cognitive impairment.

You do need to be careful with zinc supplements. Taking high-dose zinc supplements can lead to copper deficiency, which can cause anaemia, especially if you take them long term. Worse, in mice, excessive zinc supplementation actually *increases* tau phosphorylation and cognitive impairment.

We don't have any data yet that a zinc supplement for everyone is helpful. And only one of the experts I spoke to was taking it. I would work closely with your GP and a dietician to see whether you have a zinc deficiency and then take only enough supplement to get you to a healthy level without risking an overdose.

Iodine

Iodine is a nutrient that is concentrated in the thyroid. It also plays a role in supporting a healthy metabolism, as well as aiding growth and development, including brain function. The link could be the thyroid gland, where 90 per cent of your iodine is found.

A Brazilian study identified that, in men at least, having undiagnosed and untreated thyroid disease, increases your risk of dementia. The World Alzheimer Report in 2021 has called for thyroid disease to be ruled out in all people presenting with cognitive impairment. That doesn't mean iodine deficiency has been specifically linked to dementia and cognitive impairment, but indirectly it could be. Iodine deficiency is the biggest cause of thyroid problems around the world. And the biggest cause of iodine deficiency is a low-iodine diet.

How can you get more iodine in your diet? The ocean is the prime store of iodine-rich foods: kombu, kelp and wakame are common sources. Kelp contains the highest amount of iodine of any food. If you like sushi and your sushi comes wrapped in seaweed, you're probably okay. Not a fan of sushi? You might find your iodine in iodised salt.

Vitamin E

The rationale for taking vitamin E supplements to prevent and treat dementia is that this vitamin has powerful antioxidant and anti-inflammatory effects, apart from its effects on lowering cholesterol. Plus, there is some suggestion that people with Alzheimer's disease have lower blood and CSF levels of vitamin E.

It looks like diets high in vitamin E do help prevent dementia. Vitamin E is found in nuts and nut oils, pumpkin, capsicum and leafy greens. The story with vitamin E supplements is a bit different. A 2017 Cochrane review found no evidence that the vitamin helps prevent people developing dementia or slows the progression to dementia from MCI. There is no mention of taking it in midlife when your brain is healthy. Plus studies show that vitamin E supplements might increase the risk of a haemorrhagic stroke (stroke with a brain haemorrhage) by 22 per cent while lowering the risk of ischaemic stroke by only 10 per cent.

Lutein and zeaxanthin

Lutein and zeaxanthin are antioxidants that can be found in green leafy vegetables like kale, spinach, broccoli and peas. Higher levels of these antioxidants in your blood may help guard against dementia in older age.

A study published in 2022 followed over 7000 people for 26 years. It asked people about their diets, measured their blood for a whole suite of nutrients and kept doing tests to measure any cognitive decline. The study found that those participants with the highest serum levels of lutein and zeaxanthin were less likely to have dementia decades later than those with lower levels. However, in this study, a couple of things stood out to me. What people said they ate correlated very poorly with what their blood levels of key nutrients actually revealed. Which absolutely reflects my experience in my practice.

The other thing was the fact that blood levels of lycopene (the red pigment in tomatoes and pomegranates), beta-carotene and vitamins C and E didn't predict any measure of brain health at all.

There is simply no evidence for taking lutein and zeaxanthin as supplements. But having a diet packed with the all-important leafy greens and other green veggies is a no-brainer.

Ginkgo biloba

This herb is marketed widely for improving, preventing, or delaying cognitive impairment and Alzheimer's disease.

The Ginkgo Evaluation of Memory (GEM) study was an American randomised, double-blind, placebo-controlled clinical trial of 3069 people. All the participants lived at home, were aged 72 to 96 years and were followed up for an average of 6.1 years.

Each participant was either given a 120 mg extract of ginkgo biloba twice a day or a placebo. The results were that the people on ginkgo did about the same as those on a placebo.

That said, a company-sponsored review of EGb 761, an extract of ginkgo biloba, suggests that, based on four trials: 'EGb 761 may help delay progression from MCI to dementia in some individuals'. Given the qualified finding, the company sponsorship and the GEM study findings, the marketing claims feel pretty hollow.

The gut microbiome and dementia

Your gut microbiome is made up of the trillions of bugs found in your guts. These micro-organisms, mainly comprised of bacteria, are involved in functions critical to your health and wellbeing. These bacteria live in your digestive system and they play a key role in digesting food you eat, and help with absorbing and synthesising nutrients, too. Gut bugs are involved in many other important processes that extend beyond your gut, including the regulation of your metabolism, body weight and immune system, as well as your brain function.

People with Alzheimer's have less of the bugs known as Firmicutes and Bifidobacterium, but an increase in other bugs called Bacteroidetes. This imbalance impacts on some of the inflammatory pathways in the gut and is measurable in the blood stream. It has been proposed that this changes the permeability of the gut, meaning larger molecules could potentially 'leak out' of the gut. It also seems to decrease mucus production in the gut.

When I was hosting 'Healthy Living' on the 9 Radio network, I once interviewed Wayne Markman from Symbyx, a company that manufactures infrared devices to help manage the gut microbiome for neurodegenerative conditions like Parkinson's and Alzheimer's disease. I was gobsmacked that such a thing existed! Really?

I called him the next week to chat brain health. Wayne is a businessman, not a scientist. He pointed to some studies in rodents with dementia showing that, indeed, mid-infrared (MIR) light treatment aimed at the abdomen changes the gut microbiome and improves learning and memory abilities. However, that doesn't mean it will work on humans. And if it does, we are a long way off from understanding how much light to use, how often and for how long. I'm still sceptical.

> What the experts do to maintain brain health
> ## WAYNE MARKMAN
>
> Wayne uses an infrared device on his abdomen and an infrared helmet daily. He follows a Mediterranean diet, does regular exercise and takes a daily 50 mg zinc supplement plus vitamin D.

Souvenaid™

This yoghurt-like drink took the market by storm when it was first released and then bought by Danone in 2007. Its ingredients include fish oil, phospholipids, choline, uridine monophosphate, vitamin E, vitamin C, vitamin B12, vitamin B6 and folic acid. The theory is that the various ingredients in it are actively involved in maintaining neurons and, as these are the very same nutrients that tend to be lacking in the diets of people who develop Alzheimer's disease, it can only be of benefit to supplement with it.

It's a daily drink. I found it online for $114 for a pack of 24. That is over $1700 a year, so you'd want to know it works! Sadly not.

A 2020 Cochrane review of treatment with Souvenaid looked at three randomised controlled trials with a total of 1097 participants. Two of the trials investigated the use of Souvenaid in people with dementia over a period of 24 weeks. The reviewers concluded that this drink 'probably does not reduce the risk of progression to dementia in people with prodromal (i.e. early stage) Alzheimer's disease'.

Anecdotally, I have heard that lots of neurologists and geriatricians still recommend it to people despite the lack of convincing evidence. Why? Maybe because there's nothing else they can really recommend and possibly it's 'better than nothing'.

Alcohol

I *love* my wine. It is one of my real pleasures in life. I don't like getting drunk, however. In fact, one or two glasses is generally where I tap out. When researching this book, I had to examine the possibility that my love affair with my beloved drop would have to end. In the best news from this entire project, it doesn't. Depending on the research I choose to favour, I might even see it as a virtue!

Let's start with the World Alzheimer Report 2021, from Alzheimer's Disease International. They have parsed the data from all the available research and their impressive list of authors and contributors give enormous credibility to this report. Let me quote: 'Light-to-moderate alcohol consumption (≤ 2 drinks per day in men and ≤ 1 drink per day in women) may have a protective effect against stroke, due to the higher levels of HDL cholesterol, reduced platelet aggregation, lower fibrinogen concentrations and increased insulin sensitivity and glucose metabolism.'

But what about dementia specifically? How does alcohol play into either preventing it or causing it?

In 2019, a large US trial was published in the *Journal of the American Medical Association* looking at exactly this link. The Ginkgo Evaluation of Memory (GEM) study conducted from 2000 to 2008 we talked about also measured data about the study participants' alcohol intake. The conclusion? Those who started the study with perfect cognitive health and drank between 7.1 and 14 drinks per week were 40 per cent *less* likely to get dementia across the study than those who drank less than one drink per week. It didn't help those who already had MCI at the start of the study, but it didn't make it worse either. But among those who already had some MCI at the start of the study, the ones who drank more than 14 drinks a week were 70 per cent more likely to get full blown dementia. That is that famous J-shaped curve that we often hear about with alcohol, where one to two drinks a day is better than none but more than two drinks a day starts to backfire on your health big time. We don't understand why this is the case. In this study, the type of alcohol didn't matter, so you can happily have a few beers or gins a week too. Just be careful with your pouring arm! A standard serve of vodka or other spirits should be only 30 mls. And as for beer, a schooner of full-strength equals 1.6 drinks and a can is 1.4 drinks. Check the labels and as they say, 'drink responsibly'.

Heavy alcohol abuse can have severe impacts on the brain. It is not yet known whether the alcohol affects the neurons in the brain directly or because the heavy use of alcohol leads to major deficiencies in vitamin B1 and thiamine. There is also the fact that heavy drinkers tend to have other nutritional problems as well. Korsakoff's syndrome (irreplaceable loss of memory) and Wernicke-Korsakoff syndrome (mental confusion, vision issues, coma, hypothermia, low blood pressure, and muscle coordination problems) are forms of alcohol-induced brain injury which can lead to alcohol-related dementia.

How much do you need to drink to seriously damage your brain? It's not an easy calculation. I have numerous patients who drink a *lot*. Not all get dementia. One of my patients drank two bottles of sparkling wine a day between her 50s and 60s. She was diagnosed with dementia in her early 60s (i.e. very young). But she also had poorly controlled diabetes, depression, heart disease, a poor diet, never took the medication prescribed to her and didn't exercise. Did her alcohol cause her dementia? It is *very* hard to say. Her husband has now developed mild cognitive impairment as well and he never drinks alcohol. He also has terrific general health, exercises regularly and has a better diet. There is a lot of luck in this game.

So, it seems that drinking in that low-to-moderate level of seven to 14 drinks a week looks okay to good, depending on where your brain is at when you start collecting data. It should be noted that the people in the US study were an average of 72 years old. Well, similar benefits were found in a cohort of Norwegians, who were aged 60 plus.

But my favourite study is the home-grown Dubbo Study of the Elderly. This was a longitudinal study of 2805 men and women aged 60 years plus living at home and initially free of cognitive impairment. They were first assessed in 1988 and followed for 16 years. In this study, any intake of alcohol predicted a 34 per cent lower risk of dementia. 'While excess alcohol intake is to be avoided, it appears safe and reasonable to recommend the continuation of moderate alcohol intake in those already imbibing, as well as the maintenance of physical activity . . . in the hope of reducing the incidence of dementia in future years,' the authors concluded. That's good news for us who enjoy a glass of wine at the end of the day!

Tea and coffee

I love coffee and tea. I always start the day with a couple of cups of tea before switching to coffee later in the day to help give my brain a boost. For me, tea is non-negotiable, whereas I could easily give up coffee. But what does the research say about the effects of tea and coffee on the brain?

In 2018, a meta-analysis of eight different studies was published. The authors concluded that coffee consumption made no difference to your risk of developing dementia. *But* in 2021, data from the enormous UK Biobank was more conclusive. This project is following over 360,000 people. The study looked at 11.4 years of data and here's what it found: coffee intake of two to three cups a day *or* tea intake of three to five cups per day *or* their combination intake of four to six cups a day were linked with the lowest risk of stroke and dementia. Read that again. That is a *lot* of tea and coffee. Compared with those who did not drink any tea and coffee, those who had two to three cups of coffee and two to three cups of tea per day had a 32 per cent lower risk of stroke and a 28 per cent lower risk of dementia.

The reason? We're not entirely sure. Coffee and tea share overlapping components like caffeine and specific flavonoids. These flavonoids have been found to protect neurons by reducing inflammation, inhibiting β-amyloid aggregation in the brain, and offering protection from cell death. Studies tell us that coffee drinkers tend to also drink tea.

If you don't like tea or coffee, don't sweat! I'd just tick your other boxes. But if you like coffee or tea, I would lean into it rather than feeling guilty.

Takeaways

- Most supplementation is a waste of money if your body is not deficient in something in particular.
- Red wine, tea and coffee, believe it or not, are the only supplements with real evidence behind them as being beneficial for the brain.
- Omega-3 supplements can be useful if a person can't stomach oily fish, such as salmon or sardines.
- The gut biome plays an important role in the prevention of dementia.
- People who drank four to six cups of coffee or tea or a combination of both a day actually had a lower chance of having a stroke or getting dementia than those who did not drink any at all.

CHAPTER 7

Get that check-up! It could make all the difference

I did want to talk about your general health. That's because US data shows that almost half of all US adults aged 45 and older have risk factors for dementia that could be easily reversed. Not doing so is a massive missed opportunity.

You now know that looking after your brain translates pretty well into looking after your heart. It seems that there is mounting evidence that when it comes to brain health, what we do to protect – or trash – our health in midlife matters more than what we do in old age. I'm definitely not saying that if you wait until 70 to overhaul your health, get fit and get a cholesterol check, that it's game over. But the best returns for your brain health are definitely when you're younger, in midlife.

With this in mind, I thought I'd go through the various health conditions you mightn't know you have unless you check them with your doctor, and how they relate to your future risk of dementia. My message is simple. Get your health checks, accept treatment for any risk factors you have, look after your body and by doing so you will be investing in your brain.

Deafness

I'm starting here because this condition, perhaps unexpectedly, has the most profound impact on your risk of dementia. More than smoking, diabetes or high blood pressure.

A massive meta-analysis of studies was done in 2017 and was later updated to include even more trials in 2020. It was published in the prestigious medical journal, *The Lancet*. It named hearing loss as the single biggest risk for cognitive impairment and dementia.

Research is ongoing as to why this is such a significant indicator of the development of dementia. The authors pointed to a small US prospective cohort study of 194 people aged on average 54 to 55 years with normal cognition. They had at least two brain MRIs, on average 19 years apart. The study found that people with midlife hearing impairment measured by audiometry had steeper temporal lobe volume loss, including in the hippocampus. The current theory is that hearing loss just reduces brain stimulation and this might be the direct cause of cognitive impairment and dementia.

So, you book in to get your hearing tested. That's easy enough, but what next?

A 25-year prospective study of 3777 people aged 65 years or older found that people who said they had hearing problems had more dementia – *except* for the ones using hearing aids. Another study of 2040 people aged over 50 years, tested every two years over a period of 18 years, found their memory deteriorated less after they started wearing hearing aids.

Man, that is pretty convincing. So that's step one. Book a hearing test and if your hearing is off, get yourself some hearing aids ASAP!

High blood pressure (AKA hypertension)

Blood pressure is the pressure inside your arteries, measured in milli-metres of mercury or mmHg. The top number (or systolic blood pressure) is when your heart contracts and the bottom number (or diastolic blood pressure) is when your heart relaxes. So, you might hear that your blood pressure is 120 over 80. The current definition of hypertension (or high blood pressure) is systolic blood pressure of 130 mmHg or more and/or diastolic blood pressure over 80 mmHg.

There is no doubt about it, having high blood pressure is bad for you. Hypertension increases the risk of strokes, heart attacks, heart failure, atrial fibrillation and premature death. These risks increase the higher your blood pressure goes (anything starting from systolic blood pressures as low as 115 mmHg). Hypertension is also the number one modifiable risk factor for vascular dementia.

The jury is in and we now have robust evidence that hypertension is linked to cognitive decline later in life. And the biggest risk is having high blood pressure in your midlife. A 2017 study found an extra 20 per cent increase in risk of dementia for every 10 mmHg rise in systolic blood pressure during midlife. That is *massive*! Unfortunately, we are still trying to work out how it causes so much brain damage.

New research has taught us that hypertension disrupts the neuro-vascular unit, which then causes a mismatch between the energy demands of busy neurons and the delivery of oxygen and glucose from the blood stream. It seems that the blood vessels simply can't dilate in response to higher brain demand. This might be what causes some low-grade chronic inflammation in the brain that we see in mice with constantly high blood pressure.

Until recently, we weren't entirely sure what your systolic and diastolic blood pressure values should be to best protect your cognitive function. Observational studies have shown that treating high blood pressure helps reduce cognitive decline. The Systolic Blood Pressure Intervention Trial (SPRINT) hypothesised that using intensive measures to reduce blood pressure (BP) to a systolic (top number) target of less than 120 mmHg would reduce heart disease outcomes and death more than the previous standard of less than 140 mmHg. However, the trial ended up stopping early, because the benefits of more aggressively targeting lowering systolic BP below 120 were so obvious that it was deemed unethical to continue advocating the standard systolic BP of 140 mmHg.

The SPRINT Memory and Cognition in Decreased Hypertension (SPRINT MIND) study took a subset of 2800 SPRINT participants to see whether these same aggressive targets would also reduce the risk of developing dementia or mild cognitive impairment. It was a hard yes again. In the group with the aggressive BP targets, new cases of MCI were 19 per cent lower, and the rates of dementia were 15 per cent lower. A subset of these SPRINT MIND folks also had brain MRIs and the ones with the more aggressive lower BP targets showed better blood flow in their brain, especially in those with a history of cardiovascular disease.

The take-away is that we should be shooting for a systolic BP (the top number) of less than 120 mmHg rather than the more old-school 140 mmHg. And while this is critical at any age, high blood pressure needs to be sorted out in midlife for the biggest brain benefits. So, book a check-up with your GP, get your blood pressure measured and any hypertension managed. There will be other things to check out . . . keep reading!

Strokes

Having a stroke *doubles* your risk of dementia.

In 2018 the World Health Summit was convened to bring together academics, policymakers, heads of pharmaceutical and device industries, and entrepreneurs to focus on the UN's sustainable developmental goals under the leadership of the World Health Organization. Before this summit, a specialised group researching the interaction of stroke and dementia and trying to prevent them happening together gathered in Berlin to highlight what is known and what needs to be done next. The result of their findings, the Berlin Manifesto, was published in 2019.

'Stroke and dementia confer risks for each other and share some of the same, largely modifiable, risk and protective factors. In principle, 90 per cent of strokes and 35 per cent of dementias have been estimated to be preventable. Because a stroke doubles the chance of developing dementia and stroke is more common than dementia, more than a third of dementias could be prevented by preventing stroke,' the authors declared.

If mice have a stroke, their brains generate an enormous amount of inflammation and we know what that does. For a refresher head to Chapter 2 on dementia.

Diabetes

Type 2 diabetes mellitus affects 9 per cent of people in the world. Diabetes occurs when the pancreas stops producing the hormone insulin in the right amounts to help move any sugar (glucose) from the blood to the cells, which use it for fuel. When this happens the excess sugar is stored in the blood and when these levels get too high (i.e. a blood sugar spike) this can cause damage to the body's internal organs and functions. When the pancreas stops producing the right amount of insulin, that is called insulin resistance. This is generally a precursor to developing full blown diabetes. So what causes insulin resistance? In type 2 diabetes, it is usually caused by lifestyle, having too much body fat, especially around the middle, and not enough physical activity. People with type 1 diabetes are born with a pancreas that just does not produce enough insulin to move blood sugars to the cells.

People with diabetes suffer from more blindness, more small nerve damage (especially in the feet) and more kidney damage, as well as heart disease, strokes and problems with blood supply to the feet and legs. A meta-analysis of 28 prospective observational studies found that people with type 2 diabetes are 73 per cent more likely to get dementia, 56 per cent more likely to get Alzheimer's disease and 127 per cent more likely to be diagnosed with vascular dementia.

What's messy is that all the factors that make diabetes more likely to develop in someone are also risk factors for dementia. We know that insulin resistance underpins diabetes. And brain scans of patients with dementia often show patchy areas in the brain where there is reduced glucose metabolism. Many researchers have postulated that insulin resistance within the brain might drive the development of Alzheimer's disease, with many calling it brain-specific 'type 3 diabetes'.

Is it the diabetes that causes the dementia or are they both diseases of poor lifestyle and so often crop up together? That's particularly important when looking at trials of anti-diabetic medications for the prevention of dementia or to stop it from getting worse.

And those trials are a bit of a mixed bag, to be honest. The authors of a 2017 Cochrane review of seven randomised controlled trials concluded: 'We found no good evidence that any specific treatment or treatment strategy for type 2 diabetes can prevent or delay cognitive impairment.' In fact, a couple of trials for some diabetic medicines found they could make cognitive impairment worse.

I wanted to say a quick word about metformin, which is the most popular 'first line' medications to treat diabetes. If you remember the chapter on supplements, Professor David Sinclair from Harvard University takes it every day (although his aim is longevity not cognitive health specifically). I was intrigued to read the findings from a Canadian study published in 2020. The study followed 2000 people with diabetes taking various medications over time. Here's what they found: among the diabetics who had normal cognitive test results at the start of the study, those taking metformin did better on memory tests when measured after two weeks and again after two years than people taking other diabetic drugs – all of which didn't affect memory performance either way. (With the exception of a group of drugs called Sulfonylureas that can cause low blood sugar as a side effect. The memories of the participants taking this got worse over time.)

As part of the same study, the authors looked at people specifically carrying the APOE gene. Those who took a diabetes drug class called DPP4 inhibitors had a much slower cognitive decline than non-carriers. But strangely, metformin didn't give any cognitive benefits to this group with the APOE gene.

The bottom line is: if you have diabetes, you're going to need a treatment. Maybe you would choose metformin, especially if you don't carry the APOE gene. If you do have that gene, you might opt for a DPP4 inhibitor. But mostly you want to have a great diet, one that includes lots of healthy veggies, fruit, wholegrains and lean protein foods, and as little junk food and soft drink as possible. Plus, you really ought to increase your exercise, sleep well and control your blood pressure and cholesterol.

Pre-diabetes

Some people have a high blood sugar level, but not high enough to be called diabetes. These people are considered to have pre-diabetes. In 2021, a study of data from the UK Biobank cohort based on 500,000 people aged 40–69 years followed up for eight years showed this condition is also a risk for dementia. Compared to those with normal blood sugar levels, people with pre-diabetes had a 42 per cent higher risk of cognitive impairment over an average of four years and were 54 per cent more likely to develop vascular dementia (but not Alzheimer's disease) over an average of eight years.

The study suggests that if you are diagnosed with pre-diabetes, don't wait before trying to turn that ship around. Start aggressively managing it with diet, exercise and possibly medication.

High cholesterol

Observational data about the link between high cholesterol and dementia have actually been a bit mixed, with some studies finding a strong link and others finding no link at all. When it comes to relating high cholesterol to developing dementia, it is hard to separate high cholesterol from other risk factors, like, for example, high blood pressure.

In 2021, a massive British study of almost two million people found that having high LDL (AKA your bad) cholesterol in midlife (before 65 years) is modestly associated with dementia risk more than 10 years later. We're talking a 5 per cent increased risk. The researchers didn't see the same thing in older people, so it looks like once again the time to act is when you're in midlife.

Don't ignore your cholesterol. Most specialists agree that high cholesterol will contribute to your overall health in old age and here's why: good cardiovascular health leads to better cognitive health.

Your genes matter, too. Studies have linked high cholesterol with worsening cognition, specifically among APOE e4 gene carriers (especially if they have cardiovascular disease).

So it's worth getting a cholesterol level check as part of your standard blood test in midlife. But what do you do with the results? To be honest, the data is a bit mixed. There is a clear link in epidemiological and observational studies between taking a cholesterol-lowering medication called a statin and a lower risk of developing dementia, especially Alzheimer's disease. But there are conflicting results for vascular dementia. Which I find a bit weird. But wait . . . it gets weirder! Despite the promising data, results from clinical trials have been frankly disappointing and they have failed to provide any good evidence for the benefit of statin therapy in reducing the risk of dementia.

Lp(a) is another type of 'bad' cholesterol. Pronounced 'lipoprotein little a', Lp(a) can clog up your arteries, causing heart attacks and strokes. People with elevated Lp(a) are two to four times more likely to have heart attacks and strokes than people with normal Lp(a) levels. But, ironically, while having high Lp(a) blood levels increases the risk of dementia in APOE e4 carriers, it consistently lowers it in non-carriers, according to large studies.

We don't know why this is exactly, although it could be that people with this issue are often taking statins to protect them against heart attacks and strokes, especially if their cholesterol is high, and that is what protects them. You can get your blood tested for this marker, but at this point it's for interest only. Although there are several promising new treatments currently being trialled, we have no treatment for high Lp(a) at the moment, and even diet and exercise doesn't help.

But research tells us that for the people who need them, statins can cut your risk of a heart attack or stroke in half. And if you do have a heart attack or stroke, being on a statin lowers your need for surgery, stents, and your risk of dying from your heart attack. The higher your cardiovascular risk, the greater the benefit of the statin. Personally, my cardiologist found that I have high levels of Lp(a), and as early onset of heart disease and strokes runs strongly through my family, I was prescribed a statin when I turned 50.

Obesity

There is no doubt that being overweight or obese increases your risk of dementia, apart from the other health problems that come with carrying too many kilos.

A 2020 US study of 5000 people found a link between dementia risk and higher body mass index (or BMI) earlier in life for both women and men. Women who, according to their BMI, were 'overweight' in early adulthood were 1.8 more likely to get dementia. And women who were 'obese' in early adulthood were 2.45 times more likely to get dementia. A separate 2020 *Lancet* meta-analysis found that obesity in *midlife* upped the risk of dementia by 60 per cent.

On the flip side, the relationship between being overweight or obese in *later* life seemed to reduce the risk. That's actually the same thing we see in prior research.

In midlife and carrying a few too many kilos? Head to chapter 5 for some ways to tweak your diet while you look to shred!

Smoking

Smokers are at higher risk of dementia than non-smokers and people who smoke two packs a day or more in midlife *double* their risk of dementia over their lifetime.

Stopping smoking, even when you're older, reduces your risk of dementia. In one study of 50,000 men aged older than 60 years, stopping smoking for more than four years significantly reduced the risk of developing dementia over the next eight years. But it might not be *your* smoking that is the issue. Around the world, 35 per cent of non-smoking adults and 40 per cent of children are exposed to second-hand smoke. One study of women 55–64 years of age found that second-hand smoke exposure was linked to worse memory deterioration, and the greater the second-hand smoke exposure, the higher the risk.

It's never too late to stop smoking. See your GP for some help dropping the habit and you can reinvest the enormous amounts of money you will save into picking up some new hobbies to stimulate and thus improve your brain health.

Sleep-disordered breathing (SDB)

Sleep-disordered breathing (including sleep apnoea) happens when your sleep is punctuated by longer-than-normal pauses in breathing. If you do a formal sleep study these pauses in breathing are often accompanied by a significant drop in your blood oxygen levels. We see this issue in a whopping 60 per cent of elderly people. Moderate to severe sleep-disordered breathing affects 25 per cent of older men.

Does it affect the brain? Yes. The two biggest studies were both done in elderly people. One looked at women with an average age of 82 at the start of the study, and the finding revealed that SDB upped the risk of dementia by 80 per cent. More specifically, it was the degree of oxygen desaturation that was the biggest predictor of cognitive loss, rather than how loud these women snored or how many apnoeic episodes they had. Relevant? Maybe. The other study was of elderly men with an average age of 76 at the start of the study. Again, it was the oxygen desaturation that contributed to cognitive decline over time. Those men with 1 per cent or more of their sleep time spent with (blood oxygen) saturation below 90 per cent had over 1.5 times the annual decline scores in their cognition.

What we don't know is whether having sleep apnoea in midlife is as bad for your brain. I wouldn't risk it. I'd get it diagnosed and treated.

I have spent more time in Chapter 9 discussing sleep apnoea in detail, including the diagnosis and treatment. But as a general rule of thumb, if you snore, wake up tired, tend to be hot and sweaty at night or are putting on more weight than you think you should be given your diet and exercise, *please* get checked out.

Thyroid disease

A British study found that many people in clinics for frailty and/ or cognitive impairment had undiagnosed underactive or over-active thyroid glands. As previously mentioned in Chapter 6, the World Alzheimer Report 2021 has called for thyroid disease to be ruled out in all people presenting with cognitive impairment. This is because there might be a simple fix that – if resolved – would fix the cognitive impairment immediately.

But it seems having thyroid disease actually increases your risk of dementia by itself. A massive 2021 Danish study found anywhere from 10 to 20 per cent increased the risk of dementia among people who developed an underactive thyroid, especially if they didn't receive any treatment for it. Please get yours checked and if your thyroid is underactive, take your medicine!

Gum disease

Your mouth is home to over 700 species of bacteria, including some that can cause periodontal (gum) disease. Mild gum disease is called gingivitis and it starts off when bacteria accumulate in tooth plaque from a combo of food and inadequate brushing. These bacteria cause inflammation and can even lead to receding gums and bleeding. If it progresses further, you can end up with the more serious form of gum disease known as periodontitis, which can leave you with gum abscesses and loose teeth that can even fall out. Beyond bleeding gums when you're cleaning your teeth, you might experience sore gums and bad breath. Okay, none of this is good on its own, but what's the link to dementia?

Periodontitis gives you more than halitosis and tooth loss. It has been linked to diabetes, cardiovascular disease, and rheumatoid arthritis, as well as mouth and gastrointestinal cancers. A recent

US study found that the same bacteria that cause gum disease are also associated with the development of Alzheimer's disease and vascular dementia. It seems that the bacteria and the inflammatory molecules they stimulate can travel from the mouth through the bloodstream to the brain. Many of these bacteria produce toxic proteins that have been shown to actually *increase* the amount of both β-amyloid and tau protein in the brain.

The study looked at data from the National Health and Nutrition Examination Survey (NHANES), a large population study. There were 6000 people included in the study, and all had dental examinations and blood tests and were followed to see who developed dementia.

The researchers looked for the appearance of antibodies against 19 specific oral bacteria for an association with dementia. They looked for the antibodies, because if the bacteria *was* growing, it was easier to detect by looking at the body's immune response, (the development of antibodies) rather than trying to look for the bacteria itself. Of the 19 bacteria, it was *Porphyromonas gingivalis* (*P. gingivalis*) that was found to be the most common culprit for causing gum disease.

The researchers then reported that people with signs of gum disease at the first visit were more likely to go on to develop Alzheimer's disease during the study period. Importantly both Alzheimer's diagnoses and deaths were associated with the development and appearance of antibodies against *P. gingivalis*.

Another large US study published in 2020 found that having gum disease gave people a 20 per cent higher chance of developing either mild cognitive impairment or dementia.

Current clinical treatments for periodontal disease are pretty intense and expensive. Despite this, they often fail to halt periodontal disease progression. So, research for a vaccine against the *P. gingivalis* bacteria is underway. Watch this space. It's coming!

Meanwhile, you need to brush and floss twice daily. Replace your toothbrush when the bristles start splaying, or go for an electric toothbrush, and see a dentist every six months. Call now to make that appointment!

COVID-19 and the brain

Every day in my practice I have been seeing people with symptoms of long COVID-19, including brain fog. A UK study comparing before and after MRI scans of patients with COVID-19 found that parts of the brain can be affected 20 weeks after they caught the virus. People who'd had COVID-19 had a reduction in their grey matter thickness in the frontal cortex and a part of the brain next to the hippocampus. They also had evidence of tissue damage in parts of the brain responsible for their sense of smell. They had a reduction in global brain size and did worse on cognitive testing 15 weeks after catching COVID-19. This was regardless of whether they had been hospitalised or not.

Cognitive neurologist Dr Trevor Chong says the findings are concerning but if they go back to normal, they might not be an issue long-term. 'I don't think anyone knows, it's all new,' he said. He added that lockdowns endured by people during the pandemic also had deleterious effects on people's brain health by impacting their mental health, circadian rhythms, sleep and exercise. 'There could be a group of people in their mid to late 60s for whom [the effect of lockdowns] could tip them over the edge [into dementia],' he said.

Regardless, if my patients are anything to go by, while some of them are 100 per cent fine after catching COVID-19, many aren't. I'm still doing everything I can to avoid getting it. So far so good!!

I do have a GP myself, as well as a cardiologist, but I also have a blood pressure machine sitting on my desk. I have a sneaky check around once a month or so. With a family history chock-full of nasty chronic diseases, I'll be closely watching my results with my GP and attending to anything that crops up, sooner rather than later.

Make 3 appointments today:

1. Contact your GP for a blood pressure, cholesterol, thyroid and blood sugar check, a referral for a sleep study if you think that's an issue and discuss giving up smoking if you're a smoker.
2. Go to a hearing clinic to get your hearing checked.
3. Visit your dentist to get a dental check and have your teeth cleaned.

Your midlife period is the time to act for most things. There is never a bad time to iron out any health kinks you have but sooner is better!

Trevor tries to eat a generally healthy diet, without sticking to a dogmatic regime. He doesn't eat much meat or refined processed food. He sticks to the recommended 10 standard drinks a week and spreads them evenly across Friday, Saturday and Sunday nights. During the pandemic his gym membership was put on hold and he bought some exercise equipment to use at home every night for 30 minutes. He tries to protect his sleep, his young kids permitting!

Trevor is proactive in going to the GP and plans to monitor and then aggressively treat any vascular risk factors that may emerge. He takes no supplements, citing insufficient evidence.

Takeaways

- US data shows that almost half of all US adults aged 45 and older have risk factors for dementia that could be easily reversed. Not doing so is a massive, missed opportunity.
- A surprising indicator of possible dementia progression is deafness.
- Other risk factors that can be modified include obesity, diabetes, gum disease, blood pressure, thyroid issues, sleep apnoea and cholesterol.
- COVID-19 has been shown to affect some parts of the brain but it is too soon to tell if the effect is permanently deleterious. The effect of lockdowns on people's mental health also has to be considered.

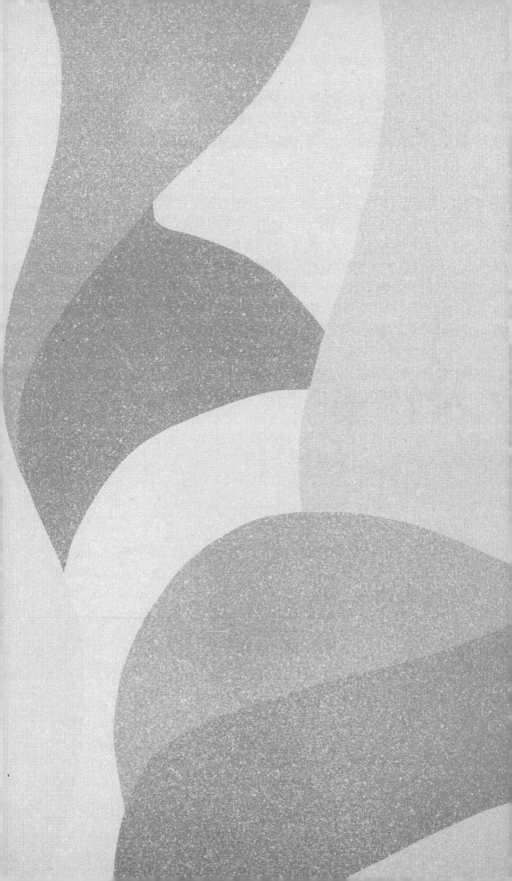

CHAPTER 8

Is depression an early indicator of dementia?

Dementia and depression can be so intertwined that when diagnosing either condition in older people it can be hard to tease them apart. Dementia is depressing and depression predisposes you to dementia.

Multiple studies have examined the link between depression and dementia. The results vary but, on the whole, late-life depression gives you a two- to five-fold increased risk of dementia. And depression in earlier life (defined as before age 60) is associated with a two- to five-fold risk of developing dementia.

What's the dementia–depression link?

We first met Professor Ian Hickie in the Introduction. Co-director of the Brain and Mind Centre at Sydney University, he is an internationally renowned researcher in clinical psychiatry. He insists that the first thing we need to challenge is our notion of exactly what depression is. 'Depression is *not* a psychological response to a hard life,' he told me. 'That would suggest there's nothing physiological going on. Depression is a multisystem disease involving the brain, and the consequences of that are hormonal, immunological and metabolic.' Think about that for a while. So many people feel that depression is a manifestation of not coping with life or having defective coping strategies. That sort of victim-blaming thinking will mean you might never overcome depression.

When it comes to the relationship between dementia and depression, Professor Hickie says there are two theories. The first is that depression is a symptom of a brain problem. 'Are they both consequences of vascular disease, where depression is the first sign of the process but over time it progresses, and the signs are more and more cognitive?' he wonders. He says that depression can emerge five to 10 years before the first cognitive signs reveal themselves in the disease process.

Indeed, a 2004 study seemed to support this when it found that people who get depression when they're already suffering from mild cognitive impairment are at more than twice the risk of developing dementia, especially Alzheimer's disease, as those without depression. Patients with depression, but who have a poor response to antidepressants are at an especially increased risk of developing dementia, which in all likelihood reinforces depression being a manifestation of a multisystem disease involving the brain.

But the second theory is that depression itself damages the brain. And Professor Hickie says there is lots of evidence that this is true. Certainly MRI studies show shrinkage of parts of the brain, such as prefrontal cortex and amygdala, in patients with depression. 'There's a view out there that depression isn't harming the brain,' Professor Hickie says. 'It is.'

The imperative to aggressively treat depression in midlife to protect the brain from subsequent cognitive decline is as important as the imperative to treat vascular risk factors such as hypertension and diabetes. We know that antidepressant medication is not just a symptom reliever but also what we call a neuroregenerative. It helps grow more brain cells, specifically in the hippocampus. Other ways to manage depression involve lifestyle changes, managing your sleep and circadian rhythms. 'You have to have a whole health approach to depression,' Professor Hickie says. So, if you care about preserving your brain's cognitive performance, preventing and aggressively treating depression in midlife is critical.

Interested? Read on!

Helping you wrangle your mental health into line

I spoke to psychologist Dr Tim Sharp for some help on this one. Tim has three degrees in psychology (including a PhD) and an impressive record as an academic, clinician and coach. He is the founder of The Happiness Institute, Australia's first organisation devoted solely to enhancing happiness in individuals, families and organisations.

I asked Tim to share his top tips for protecting our mental health in midlife. He gave me several and was very keen to point out that they are in no particular order. He also insisted that I tell you that you don't have to do *all* of them. Treat them like an all-you-can-eat mental health buffet. Experiment, play around with what works for you. 'Make your own recipe,' Dr Sharp suggests. 'Different strategies will work for different people.'

With this in mind, I give you Dr Tim's tips.

1. Exercise

'Most people think about exercise for its physical benefits, but exercise is one of the best stress-busters and antidepressants we have,' Dr Sharp says. It's something I talk about all the time with my patients who have depression.

It's thought that exercise causes the blood vessels to open up, including those supplying the brain. Exercise is also thought to affect the link between the hypothalamus, the pituitary and adrenal glands – also known as the HPA axis – and, thus, on your reactions to stress. Other theories include simple distraction and social interaction.

There are so many health benefits from regular exercise:

- improved sleep
- increased interest in sex
- better endurance

- stress relief
- improvement in mood
- increased energy and stamina
- reduced tiredness that can increase mental alertness
- weight reduction
- reduced cholesterol and improved cardiovascular fitness.

WHICH EXERCISE?

Aerobic exercises, including jogging, swimming, cycling, walking, gardening and dancing, have been specifically studied for mood disorders and proven to reduce both anxiety and depression. Tim does a combo of high intensity and walking, especially bushwalking, which combines both exercise and getting into nature (see Tip 2) for him.

2. Connect with nature

These days I feel like I either sit all day in my windowless surgery or in front of a screen, typing. I live such an urban existence, but I hadn't realised the risk this posed to my mental health. Tim suggests countering our screen-based existence by heading into nature. 'When I'm in the bush, I just feel so much better,' Tim told me. 'Being in green, around trees and away from screens has lots of benefits.'

Research backs him up here. The sounds of nature have been shown to help recovery from stress. Group walks in nature have been linked with significantly lower depression and stress, as well as better mental wellbeing. Even gardening has been shown to be a stress-buster.

3. Practise self-compassion

Before you roll your eyes, read the science! Self-compassion is a positive psychological tool where you extend compassion to yourself, often during periods of suffering. We women are *terrible* at it. We are often totally amazing at practising compassion for others but trying to direct it back at ourselves leaves us feeling like an idiot. It sounds a lot like self-pity, or being self-serving, self-indulgent or self-centred, right?

But what if it turns out that practising self-compassion could protect your mental health, your heart and your brain as well? Interested now? Well, I was fascinated by a study published in 2022 by Rebecca Thurston, Professor of Psychiatry at University of Pittsburgh. Her study looked at 195 women with an average age of 59 years, free of cardiovascular disease. They went through a battery of physical tests as well as tests to assess their self-compassion. Those who tested higher on self-compassion were associated with lower thickness of their coronary arteries – a measure of vascular disease. This persisted regardless of the measures of blood pressure, weight, sugar levels and even depression scores.

In other words, being compassionate towards yourself reduces your odds of a heart attack. Professor Thurston said it makes sense that it would be protective against dementia, too. Because what's good for the heart is good for the brain.

Tim pointed me to the work of his colleague, Dr Kristin Neff from University of Texas at Austin. 'Having compassion for oneself is really no different than having compassion for others,' Dr Neff says. To have compassion for others you need to notice that they are suffering, she says. After noticing the suffering, you need to be moved so that your heart responds with warmth, caring and the desire to help. Showing understanding and kindness to others when they fail or make mistakes, rather than judging them harshly, is a big part of it. Finally, when you feel compassion for someone, you understand that it's a shared experience. We all make mistakes.

Self-compassion means directing all of that at yourself. Instead of just trying to ignore your own pain or tell yourself to get over it, you acknowledge that things are tough at the moment. Ask yourself: how can I comfort and care for myself in this moment?

But how do you create self-compassion?

Tim suggests three steps that might help:

- **Mindfulness.** That means being aware and acknowledging how you're thinking and feeling at the moment and being accepting of the experience itself.
- **Self-kindness.** 'Treat yourself as well as you treat your friends,' Dr Tim suggests.
- **Understanding and connectedness.** As Dr Tim explains, it's normal to have negative thoughts and emotions, but through our connectedness to and understanding of others, we realise that other people have these negative thoughts too. It turns out we're not alone!

4. Prioritise good nutrition

'If you feed yourself rubbish, your body's not going to work as well and your brain's not going to work as well [as they could],' Tim explains. Multiple studies have shown that the relationship between your diet and your risk of poor mental health is linear. The worse your diet, the higher the risk of depression. The mechanism? It seems that the worse your diet, the more disrupted your gut microbiome and the higher the levels of inflammation generated in the body. This directly leads to immune system disruption in the gut and translates to more immune system issues in general, including inflammation of the brain.

The link between junk food and immune dysfunction is probably at least in part a disrupted gut microbiome. We have mentioned the importance of this previously. This complex ecosystem of microbes weighs around 1 kg, which is similar to the weight of the brain. Your gut microbiome is made up of trillions of micro-organisms (10^{14} to be exact), which is greater than the number of cells in your body! In a healthy person three-quarters of these bacteria are Firmicutes and Bacteroides. As scientific methods have improved, allowing us to study them properly, we have worked out that these bugs are *essential* for our bodies to work, principally by managing our immune systems. They also make us some essential nutrients such as vitamins K, B2, B9 and B12, as well as tryptophan (which is the precursor to serotonin, the so-called calming hormone), all of which are essential for brain health.

What the experts do to maintain brain health
PROFESSOR REBECCA THURSTON

Rebecca's priority is her sleep, which she has struggled with from time to time. When insomnia hits, she uses CBT-I (cognitive behavioural therapy for insomnia) on herself but doesn't restrict any sleep. She exercises six days a week doing either cardio, strength training, yoga or online HIITS. She practises mindfulness meditation most days (time varies), is social and sticks pretty closely to a Mediterranean diet. She takes a multivitamin plus a vitamin D supplement.

SHOULD YOU JUST HAVE A PROBIOTIC TO BOOST YOUR MOOD?

No! There is no evidence probiotics work in this way. Perhaps that's because your stomach pumps all your food through a hydrochloric acid bath designed to kill off all the bacteria it meets. In fact, we still don't know how much, if any, probiotics from supplements even survive the journey through the stomach to make it to the large intestine, which is where the key microbiome players live. Also, most probiotic supplements only have one or two strains of probiotics. But eating the right foods can encourage multiple healthy strains of probiotics to grow.

You can get some of your probiotics from fermented foods such as pickles, kimchi and fermented milk products like kefir. These are all high in probiotics but also contain important nutrients such as fibre and antioxidants.

5. Set and move towards meaningful goals

While this might sound a bit daunting, it is actually quite simple. It just means 'something that gives us a reason to get out of bed in the morning, a positive focus,' Dr Tim explains. Luckily, there is no right and wrong on this one. If you're thinking that not being a warrior for climate change mitigation has doomed your brain to an early demise, think again. Dr Tim says that a meaningful goal for you could be something as simple as 'getting fitter or stronger or it could be career-focused. As long as you're setting and moving towards a goal'.

This fits perfectly for someone like me. I always have a hundred projects on the hop, such as cooking, researching and writing this book, reading my way through the classics, and staying in touch with friends and family. But what about people who are a tad more relaxed in life? Maybe put some thought towards the things that you like about your life and want more of. Then start thinking about practical ways you can make them happen.

6. Get enough sleep

'I've been banging on about this for 20 years,' Tim says. There is such a strong association between sleep problems and depression (97 per cent of people with depression report some major and often distressing sleep issues), that some researchers have suggested that depression can't be diagnosed in someone who is sleeping well. It looks like the brain changes that happen with depression interfere with sleep. But sleep issues cause depression, too.

Almost 30 years ago now, the National Institute of Mental Health Epidemiologic Catchment Area study interviewed 8000 people on two occasions, one year apart. The researchers found that people who had insomnia at the first interview were much more likely to have gone on to develop depression a year later. Subsequent studies have confirmed that when it comes to sleep and depression, the relationship is bidirectional, and the tail wags the dog as much as the dog wags the tail.

For tips on getting enough sleep, head to Chapter 9.

7. Have good quality relationships

'If you look at all the literature, positive relationships that give you a sense of belonging and connectedness are protective of your mental health,' Dr Tim said. 'Friendships are super important. You just need one or two people who you can trust.' This can include your intimate partner, of course.

What makes a solid connection? Sure, it's about having someone who has your back and supports you when the chips are down. 'But supporting and giving is as important as receiving,' Dr Tim insists.

If a relationship is solid, invest in it and nurture it. Especially your intimate partner. It's easy for a solid relationship to lose its potency out of negligence. 'One of the most common traps is neglect and taking the other person for granted,' Dr Tim warns. He suggests prioritising the relationships that matter most and actively expressing love and gratitude. 'What did you used to do for your partner when you first started dating?'

For some couples, Tim says, they just naturally continue to love and cherish one another, and it comes easily. For others, it takes work. 'If we look at the happiest couples, they argue as much as the unhappy couples, but they make up more quickly and forgive more easily.' They're things we can all improve on, Dr Tim says.

So hopefully if you do have poor mental health, especially with a nastier condition like dementia, you have been convinced to get it sorted. Where do you start?

Psychological therapies for depression

Otherwise known as 'talking therapies', psychological therapies are hugely important. Experts recommend that they should be undertaken by everyone with depression, whether antidepressant medicine is being used or not. All these therapies involve talking about your thoughts with a professional to better understand your own thinking and behaviour as well as to resolve your problems. Ultimately the goal is to reduce your depressive symptoms and improve your life.

Some commonly used psychological interventions are Cognitive Behavioural Therapy (CBT), Interpersonal Therapy, Mindfulness, Commitment and Acceptance Therapy, and Supportive Psychotherapy.

What the experts do to maintain brain health
DR TIM SHARP

Tim likes to exercise, something he does five to six days a week. He eats well and checks in with his GP once a year to keep his body in shape.

Tim has publicly discussed his lifelong battles with depression. As the guru in combatting it, he practises what he preaches for himself. This includes meditating daily and avoiding spending a lot of time on his mobile phone. 'I do these strategies even in the good times,' he told me. So, when it [depression] does come back, it won't come back so badly.'

Cognitive behavioural therapy

CBT is based on the idea that our emotions are simply a result of our thoughts. It aims to help you challenge your unhelpful 'head-talk', which is the stuff we tell ourselves every day, and to understand that just because we might feel something, doesn't necessarily mean it is true. For example, you might say to yourself: 'Why would I bother going on that date? – it's going to be a disaster anyway.' This not only makes you feel depressed and anxious about it, but you unconsciously bring that energy to the date, and guess what? It is a disaster!

In CBT, your psychologist or therapist will challenge you to come up with the evidence for your negative head-talk and then to consider the evidence against it. It helps you challenge your thoughts and become a bit more balanced in your thinking.

CBT has good evidence for managing anxiety and depression.

INTERPERSONAL PSYCHOTHERAPY

This style of therapy is focused on resolving interpersonal problems that are causing issues like depression. The therapy is usually time limited (three to four months) and provides tools to help people manage communication in difficult relationships. Because while depression isn't always caused by a problematic relationship, it can affect relationships if you withdraw from those you love or become a bit obsessed. It shouldn't be the mainstay of your therapy, but it might be helpful to resolve some grief, or transition into a new state (from married to divorced, for example), or explore a problematic relationship/s.

This type of therapy has good evidence for treating depression but also for treating eating disorders, drug and alcohol use, and even bipolar disorder.

MINDFULNESS

Mindfulness is a therapy aimed at getting you to focus on the present moment, rather than worrying about the past or things that haven't even happened yet. Mindfulness is an activity you can do by yourself in a quiet moment, but you might find it helpful to get taught by a therapist or even an app.

Below is my go-to mindfulness meditation activity that I pull out of the bag to use at times of peak stress. But to be really effective, I have to practise it regularly.

- Sit on a comfortable chair. Put your bottom right back in the chair. Make sure your feet are resting gently on the ground, equally weighted.
- Gently close your eyes; don't scrunch your eyelids up, just rest them very gently together.
- Relax your feet, resting them gently on the floor.
- Relax your thighs, letting them fall into the chair.
- Let your tummy blob out, no holding it all in!
- Let your shoulders drop.
- Let your hands rest comfortably on your lap.
- Relax your brow.
- Unclench your jaw.
- Now take a long, slow breath in through your nose and out again through your nose.
- As you breathe, focus your mind on the way the air feels cooler and sharper going in and warmer and softer going out.
- Just focus on the way the breath feels on the tip of your nose.
- If your mind wanders, imagine yourself gently scooping your thoughts back and placing them gently on the tip of your nose.
- Slowly focus on three distinct things you can hear. Just list them slowly in your head. It might be the traffic outside, the hum of a computer, a voice in the distance.
- Keep breathing.
- Slowly focus on three distinct things you can feel. Just list them slowly in your head. It might be the way your back feels against the chair, the way your left hand feels against your left thigh, etc.

The secret is to practise. Start with 20 minutes a day. Once you are good at it and can switch your mind off quickly, you can do it whenever you want and when you need it most. Yes! You can do a quick five minutes of mindfulness meditation when you're feeling exhausted if you can find a quiet spot to sit.

There is good evidence for mindfulness helping with depression and anxiety.

ACCEPTANCE AND COMMITMENT THERAPY

Usually referred to as ACT, this is based on the principles of mindfulness but with some fabulous additions. It is designed to help people *accept* their feelings of anxiety and *commit* to living in accordance with personal values. Practically speaking, it has three core parts. Firstly, it helps you to accept negative thoughts and emotions, and to think of them as passing through and not defining you. It also helps you to develop psychological skills to deal more effectively with those negative thoughts and emotions to reduce their impact on you. Secondly, it helps you to clarify your true values (your heart's deepest desires for how you want to live your life, how you want to treat yourself, others, and the world around you). And thirdly, it helps you use these identified values to guide and inspire your life so that you authentically live a meaningful life that makes you feel more engaged and better about yourself. It also helps you be mindful about the changes you are making and any new feelings that arise.

At its core, ACT helps you just accept what is out of your personal control and commit to action that improves and enriches your life. I *love* this therapy. I have noticed the psychologists I refer to are using it more and more and the dividends have been simply amazing for them! It has good evidence behind it in treating stress, anxiety, personality disorders and even schizophrenia.

SUPPORTIVE PSYCHOTHERAPY

This is a conversational-style therapy that aims to make you feel comfortable and less anxious, while coming up with practical ways for you to cope with stressful situations. It doesn't have a rigid structure because it might be affected by your personality (i.e. some of your character traits and natural defence mechanisms), as well as your own natural abilities, including any poor cognitive functioning, lower IQ or learning disabilities. But it has good evidence as a treatment for depression.

These aren't the only therapies around. They're just the main ones. Some practitioners also use dialectical behavioural therapy, cognitive analytical therapy, group therapy, family therapy and psychodynamic psychotherapy, amongst others. All have varying degrees of evidence as to their effectiveness. Certain psychologists have more expertise in some therapies than others and some will pick the style of therapy they think will work for you based on your personality, your symptoms and your story.

Finding your dream therapist

Lots of my patients are quite resistant to having therapy. 'I've tried it, it doesn't work,' I hear them say. Often the real problem has been a real mismatch between therapist and patient. Not every therapist will work for everyone, and you might need to kiss a lot of frogs to find your prince. I understand though, at upwards of $200 a visit, kiss too many frogs and you might feel that you will go broke looking for your perfect match!

In Australia your GP or family doctor is often the gatekeeper to a therapist. I think this system is great. I know my patients well and I also know my local therapists really well, so I feel like I can pick the right therapist for the right patient. However, I don't always get it right.

Some of my patients come in telling me that the lady at the shop or their cousin highly recommends such and such a therapist.

Just remember that what works for your friend mightn't work for you. I generally find that approach a complete waste of time.

Another thing to remember is that in any sort of supportive therapy it is super important to establish a therapeutic relationship. So it might feel like the therapist agrees that all your issues are the fault of your asshole ex or your asshole boss or your awful mum, at least for the first few sessions. But at some point, they have to help you challenge your own head-talk and start to reframe your feelings, thinking, let some ideas go, and commit to new ones. For your own good, they will need to push you out of your comfort zone. That doesn't mean they're a bad therapist or don't 'get' you. If you are going to part with your hard-earned cash and sign up for psychological therapies, I would urge you to go with a *truly* open mind and look to embrace change that will make your life better.

You also need to stick with it. If you just do two or three sessions and give up, chances are therapy won't work for you. My analogy is this: you cannot join the gym and then give up a week later because you aren't running a marathon yet. It takes time and practice.

But if this is all sounding too hard, never fear! The evidence is mounting that bypassing the personal therapist and opting for an app is a great, and definitely cheaper, option. I have listed the apps I use at the end of this chapter.

Antidepressant medications

Getting on top of your depression to help your brain may mean taking an antidepressant medication. Do they work? Yes, they really, really do. In 2018, a huge meta-analysis of trials was published in the prestigious medical journal *The Lancet*. Examining data from 116,477 patients over 522 trials, the authors found that 'all anti-depressants were more efficacious than placebo in adults with major depressive disorder'. That doesn't mean they're not without issues or that they're for everyone.

In *The Lancet* analysis, the most effective type of antidepressants for reducing depression, which were the old-school tricyclic antidepressants such as amitriptyline, norpramin and tofranil, had a very high rate of side effects, many of which were intolerable to patients. That's why, despite being very good at their job, they're not used that often. The authors found that newer SSRI antidepressants such as escitalopram, mirtazapine, paroxetine, agomelatine and sertraline had good efficacy but the least side effects.

That said, while antidepressants do work better than placebo, it's often not a *bunch* better. In 2020, the Royal Australian and New Zealand College of Psychiatrists updated their guidelines for the management of mood disorders, including depression. They concluded that nobody should have a pill chucked at them without psychological therapies added in. And for mild to moderate depression, doctors should be a bit slower to dole out the prescriptions and only keep them for people with severe symptoms or those who don't respond to lifestyle changes and psychological therapies alone.

Transcranial magnetic stimulation

In this relatively new treatment, magnetic fields, generated by a simple coil placed on your head, are used to stimulate a small and very specific area on the surface of the brain. They work by rebalancing activity across brain networks. A session of transcranial magnetic stimulation takes 10 to 30 minutes while you are wide awake and you need to have them on around 20 consecutive weekdays. While being super well tolerated, it is surprisingly effective for depression. In Australia you qualify to try it if you have had no success with multiple medications.

Complementary and alternative options for depression

Lots of my patients are really reluctant to take an antidepressant medication. They believe they are addictive (they're not) or that their depression isn't bad enough to warrant a medication. They prefer a 'natural' supplement or herbal treatment instead. So, let's take a look at the options.

Aromatherapy

I have to admit, studies are a little shaky on this but aromatherapists agree, scents really do help generate a sense of tranquillity. My patients are used to coming into my surgery where I have a bizarre mash-up of incense, candles, oil burners and reed diffusers. My partners at my surgery call my office the 'Day Spa'. Luckily, my obsession with scents has a tiny bit of grounding in science.

There have been a few small trials of various essential oils either being inhaled or used as part of a massage for help with mood swings amongst various groups of people. A recent review of studies found no randomised controlled trials at all. But the five poorer quality studies on inhalation aromatherapy and eight studies on aromatherapy massage mostly found significant antidepressive effects.

Participants in these studies reported feeling less moody and there was also a drop in their cortisol levels, measured through their saliva. Oils studied include clary sage, rosemary, lavender and bergamot. Given that there is practically no downside from aromatherapy, I'd go for whatever scent you like. Not because of the science, which is pretty weak, but because you enjoy it. I am one of those people who just loves these kinds of scents, so at any given time at home and in my surgery I tend to have one bubbling or burning away.

Studies of aromatherapy for dementia with or without depression have been pretty disappointing. But animal therapy, exercise, massage and touch therapy were all found in a recent review of studies to benefit people with dementia *and* depression.

Curcumin (*Curcuma longa*)

A 2017 meta-analysis of six trials of curcumin for depression, with a total of 377 people, found – with albeit very low quality of evidence – a small but significant short-term benefit from curcumin. Not much downside in taking this.

Light therapy

Light therapy can be used to treat forms of depression where a lack of access to sunlight is thought to be contributing to depression (like seasonal depression, where you go into a funk come wintertime). You basically sit or work near a light therapy box for about 30 minutes a day. A Cochrane review analysed the effects of light therapy given *with* antidepressants versus sham light therapy plus antidepressants on non-seasonal depression. They found a small decrease in the severity of the depression.

For patients with seasonal depression, a meta-analysis of 19 poor quality trials found using light therapy of a significant benefit. I found some light boxes online from AU$50, so not a massive outlay, and could be worth considering if you get seasonal depression.

Acupuncture

A high-quality Cochrane review meta-analysed 49 studies for acupuncture in adults with depression. The researchers found some evidence that it could be effective for depression but the quality of the trials was pretty poor, which left the authors well short of a fist-thumping endorsement. But if you can tolerate it well and it's working for you, why not?

St John's wort (*Hypericum perforatum*)

This is an ancient herb that has been around and used for brain health for hundreds of years. It appears to increase the amount of serotonin, dopamine and noradrenaline in the brain, which are all chemicals that, when depleted, are linked to both depression and anxiety. Another Cochrane review, this time from 2008, reviewed 29 studies in 5489 patients, all with mild to moderate depression, comparing the herb to placebo or standard antidepressants over four to 12 weeks. The conclusion? Massive thumbs up from Cochrane, which is unusual. The findings stated: 'The available evidence suggests that the hypericum extracts tested in the included trials:

- are superior to placebo in patients with major depression
- are similarly effective as standard antidepressants
- and have fewer side effects than standard antidepressants.'

That's a pretty compelling conclusion. Remember, it is for mild to moderate depression, which we wouldn't usually be suggesting an antidepressant for anyway, but it might be perfect if that is you.

The caveat the review highlighted was the fact that lots of commercial products are dodgy. They pointed to a German study that looked at commercially available St John's wort products, finding many of them contained only minor amounts of bioactive compounds. I'm not sure how to get around that. If your St John's wort product isn't working, try going for a different brand, which might be slightly less dodgy.

S-adenosyl methionine (SAMe)

SAMe is a compound found naturally in the body, made from homocysteine and folate. It regulates hormones and maintains cell membranes. It is commercially available in supplement form. Once again, we have a Cochrane review to draw on, this time from 2016, and comparing eight trials of around 900 adults. The studies were of very low quality and the authors were unable to support its use, calling for higher quality trials.

Omega-3 fats

A 2015 Cochrane review of 25 studies including 1400 people found a minor benefit over a placebo, but the studies were of such poor quality that the authors were reticent to give it the nod.

Massage therapy

There is some evidence from tiny trials that massage may decrease the body's stress and inflammatory responses and improve the immune function. Studies have been done on massage therapy for anxiety and depression, but you can drive a truck through the differences in methodology of the trials. However, there is no downside and if it works for you, I say go for it.

Vitamin supplements

The results for treating depression with vitamin supplementation are a mixed bag. For vitamin B6 supplements, a review of just two studies showed no benefit over placebo. For folic acid (AKA vitamin B9) supplements, a 2003 Cochrane review found that while they don't do much on their own, they might help antidepressants work better. But the small number of trials saw the researchers stop short of recommending it.

A 2014 meta-analysis of vitamin D supplements for depression, looking at seven trials, two for clinically significant depression, showed 'a moderate, statistically significant effect'. But then came the usual caveat that the studies were of poor quality and further research should be done before any firm recommendations can be made.

The perimenopause depression risk

As I am writing this, I am still (at age 54) in hard-core perimenopause and although I have never suffered from mental health issues, I feel like all my patients, as well as my friends, have suffered during this stage of life.

So, let's talk science! Perimenopause (which encompasses the menopause transition through to the first few months after menopause proper) is a 'window of vulnerability' for developing depression. This period of time constitutes the highest risk of depression in a woman's life.

For peri women – you are between two and four times more likely to experience depression than at *any other* time of your life. If you have ever had a battle with depression, you have an almost 60 per cent chance of it coming back as you hit perimenopause.

While there are tons of theories as to why, the exact mechanism remains elusive. But here is what we know so far. Risk factors for depression in perimenopause include:

- previous hormonal mood problems (postnatal depression, premenstrual syndrome, premenstrual dysphoric disorder)
- previous depression
- adverse life events or trauma
- premature menopause
- hot flushes.

Depression in perimenopause often has distinct characteristics, including a tendency towards anxiety, irritability and sleep issues. These tend to overlap with classic perimenopause symptoms.

Why hormone replacement therapy (AKA HRT) is not the best antidepressant

There is some evidence that HRT has an effect similar to that of classic antidepressant medications specifically for depressed perimenopausal women. But it's not your first cab off the rank in choice. Pauline Maki, who is professor of Psychiatry, Psychology and Obstetrics and Gynecology at the University of Illinois at Chicago and generally recognised as a world leader in the interface between menopause and the brain, says the first stop should be asking what has worked for the patient in the past. Because so many women who experience depression in midlife have been there, done that before, many know exactly what works best for them. Be that a specific medication or psychotherapy, Professor Maki says we want to use therapies that have worked before.

Dr Karen Magraith, president of the Australian Menopause Society, has a special interest in mood issues in perimenopause. She told the Australian Menopause Society that HRT 'may be particularly applicable if the patient has a history of hormone-related mood disturbance or other symptoms of perimenopause such as vasomotor symptoms (hot flushes)'.

CAN HRT PREVENT DEPRESSION FROM HAPPENING AT ALL?

Maybe! Research published in 2018 from the University of North Carolina School of Medicine showed that hormone replacement therapy during perimenopause helped to prevent the onset of depression. This study enrolled women who were around perimenopause age and who had some low levels of depressive symptoms (but not enough to be called depressed). They received either a placebo or transdermal oestradiol (that means oestrogen via a patch or a gel) and micronised progesterone (the 'safest' form of progesterone). For the women on the HRT, 17 per cent developed depression. That compared to 32 per cent of women on a placebo. The women who had the most success from the HRT-as-prevention strategy were those with 'a greater number of stressful life events in the six months preceding study enrolment'. Think divorce, job loss, etc.

Given that almost 60 per cent of women who have ever experienced depression are going to see it return in perimenopause, Professor Pauline Maki suggested in a webinar to the International Menopause Society that certain women would benefit from using HRT as a preventer. Like Dr Karen Magraith, she thinks it is particularly appropriate if the women are having some other menopause symptoms such as hot flushes and night sweats.

What about anxiety? Does it increase your risk of dementia?

I am interested in this question because anxiety as a condition is more common than depression (where the link to dementia is clear).

US data suggests anxiety is the most common mental illness in the US and is experienced by 18.1 per cent of the population every year (compared to 6.7 per cent with depression). And even though it's very treatable, less than 40 per cent of those suffering get treatment for their anxiety.

And that number only went up in the pandemic.

The relationship between anxiety and subsequent dementia isn't as clear as depression and subsequent dementia, though. A meta-analysis of six studies of older adults found that those with anxiety had a 57 per cent higher risk of developing dementia. The risk was highest in those who started experiencing anxiety when they were older, so the authors suggested that, like depression, anxiety in older adults might actually be an early sign of dementia. Then in 2021 a new US study was published that followed 1400 people aged 70 and over, over eight years. While depression strongly predicted dementia, anxiety didn't. But what about those of us in midlife?

A 2018 meta-analysis of four studies comprising almost 30,000 people did find anxiety in midlife increased the risk of dementia later in life. However, the risk wasn't huge and the study quality was poor.

The Australian Imaging, Biomarker & Lifestyle Flagship Study of Ageing (AIBL) is the largest study of its kind in Australia. Launched in 2006, its authors are seeking to discover which biomarkers, cognitive characteristics, and health and lifestyle factors predict the development of subsequent Alzheimer's disease. One of the things the study is looking at is anxiety. And the quality of this trial and its data analysis is excellent.

The results have started coming in from various studies from this major research and there certainly *does* seem to be a link between anxiety and poorer cognitive function. In 2018, a study based on the AIBL data found that the real risk factor for developing dementia was chronic anxiety, or people who live with anxiety daily. While the authors said it is too early to call anxiety out as a definite risk for dementia, chronic anxiety is unpleasant and worth trying to fix or at least ameliorate. Chat to your GP or look at the lifestyle advice on combatting depression from Dr Tim starting on page 155. All are good for anxiety as well.

Loneliness and brain health

I thought I would look at this as a separate mental health issue because the data on loneliness and cognitive ill health is interesting. In 2022, a study was published in the journal *Neurology* looking at the link between loneliness and dementia. The results weren't great for those who spend a lot of time alone. Out of the 2308 participants followed over a 10-year period (average age 73 years and 56 per cent of them women) who had no dementia at the start of the study, the dementia risk was more than 50 per cent higher for the Eleanor Rigbys of the world, compared with people who were not lonely. This followed another study of 60,000 people published just a month earlier in the journal *JAMA Network Open* which suggested that loneliness in elderly women in the US was associated with a 27 per cent higher risk for severe cardiovascular disease. And we know what is good for the heart is good for the brain.

Commenting on the *Neurology* study, Manfred Beutel, MD, director of the Clinic for Psychosomatic Medicine at the University Hospital of Mainz, Germany, pointed out that, 'just because someone is alone, it does not mean that they are lonely. Someone is only lonely if solitude is painful for them, if they feel isolated, or feel like they don't belong anywhere'.

It's hard to know whether disconnecting from community and friends is a symptom of depression which then leads to dementia or is a symptom of dementia itself. It also raises the question of whether loneliness should be targeted like treating high blood pressure. If your mum wants to be alone and really doesn't want to leave the house or catch up with her old friends, can you force her? But for us in midlife, investing in meaningful connections will do lots for our brain. The next time you really, really don't want to go to that dinner or girls' night out, make sure that avoidance isn't becoming a pattern. If it is, time for a mental health check-in with your GP or psychologist. Maybe we should all fake it till we make it and just make ourselves go?

In short

I did want to emphasise one more time that depression is not a psychological response to a hard life. It is a physical brain problem that is caused by and, importantly, causes cognitive decline. Whichever path you go down, get your mental health dealt with in midlife to optimise your future brain health.

One of my patients, Trish, was 67 when depression made an unwelcome return after she last had it in her mid-40s. Trish had a stressful job as an accountant in a big firm and she was sure this was to blame. We started with some minor lifestyle changes (although she had a lifelong problem of insomnia, there weren't too many changes she could actually make as she had a super mental-health-friendly lifestyle) and then she saw a psychologist.

She got worse. We started an antidepressant medication, to no avail. After a second failure, I sent her to a psychiatrist, who upped the doses, then changed her again, then prescribed a round of transcranial magnetic stimulation. Nothing worked. It was now two years down the track. By now Trish was apathetic, seeing very few friends and felt like her brain was just not functioning. She felt vague and like she couldn't remember things. She gave up work and I noticed she hardly left the house.

This was a woman who had done tango dancing, yoga and pilates weekly but now was doing no exercise at all. She no longer talked to me about her next trip overseas or the latest bars she had just been to with her huge circle of friends.

The psychiatrist wanted to try electroconvulsive therapy on her to try to turn the ship around. But as her cognitive symptoms caught up to and then overtook her mood symptoms, it became clear that, in Trish's case, her depression was the first sign of an impending cognitive problem.

I now have her booked in to see a neurologist. I wonder whether she got caught in a chicken-and-egg situation where her depression was both a symptom of and a contributor to her cognitive impairment? Could we have done anything else? Her physical health is awesome. She's on hardly any tablets for anything. There were so few points at which we could intervene.

I am devastated to see what is happening to this incredible woman. I know her friends and family are, too.

Takeaways

- Developing depression at any point in life can lead to a higher risk of developing dementia as you grow older. Developing depression later in life can be a sign of progressing dementia.
- Paying attention to your sleep, diet, work–life balance, relationships and stress is critical in preventing depression and, subsequently, the possibility of dementia.
- HRT can be effective for the treatment of depression, especially in perimenopausal women.
- Studies are showing that there is a link between chronic anxiety and poorer cognitive function.

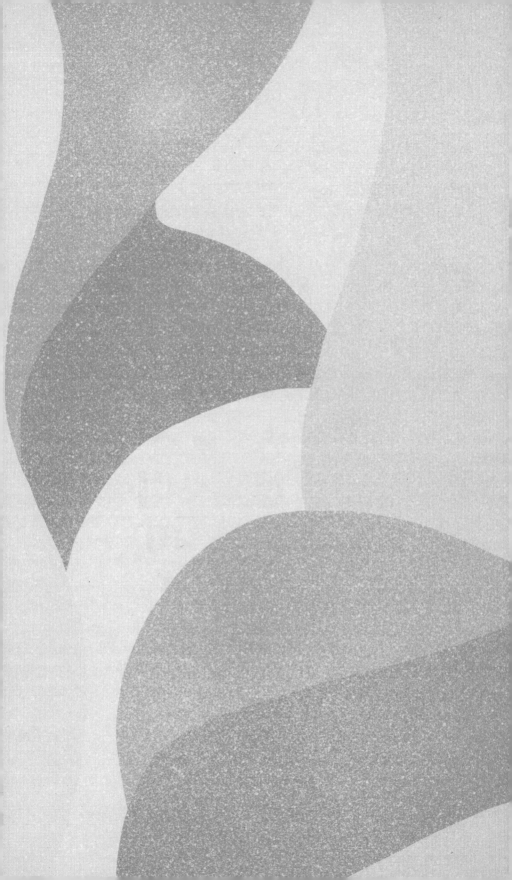

CHAPTER 9

Catching zzzzzs. Why a good night's sleep matters for dementia

I am going to 'fess up that I have been a terrible sleeper for the past few years. I used to be a gold-medal Olympian of sleep. I reckon by age 48, though, my sleeping started to go to the dogs. Now, at 54, pulling an all-nighter doesn't mean what it used to! (Until recently, the last time I have gone to bed and then just woken up six to eight hours later was some time last year!) I'm perimenopausal so I am often falling asleep exhausted, only to wake up one or two hours later and stare at the ceiling.

If I was worried about that before, writing this book has made me tackle sleep as my highest priority. Why? Sleep and cognitive decline frequently come packaged together. I was alarmed by a 2017 meta-analysis of 27 studies that found sleep problems raise the risk of cognitive impairment by 65 per cent, and that poor quality sleep could explain up to 15 per cent of Alzheimer's disease cases.

Okay, time to get serious. Let's talk sleep and work out how to wrangle yours back to health.

What is normal sleep and how does it change as you get older?

Doctors think of a good night's sleep as a night when you fall asleep reasonably easily, don't get up during the night and wake up when you're ready – not too early – feeling refreshed. Everyone can have the odd bad night but regularly struggling to fall asleep or not sleeping through the night is not normal for healthy people of any age. Sure, not everyone needs the same amount of sleep, and quality of sleep can vary with the different stages in your life. But that's the benchmark.

Technically, sleep is a state of unconsciousness in which the brain is relatively more responsive to internal than external stimuli. We think that the sleep–wake cycle serves a bit like a rechargeable battery: the brain charges during sleep and discharges when you're awake.

We used to think of sleep as a kind of passive state that happened when we withdrew sensory inputs. You stop talking, turn off the lights, it's quiet, so you sleep. We now know it's far more complex than that. For example, we know that there is a 'switch' for sleep – the ventrolateral preoptic nucleus (VLPO) in the hypothalamus. If you use an MRI machine to look at someone's brain while they sleep, this VLPO lights up (which means blood supply to this area increases) and seems to release two important chemicals: GABA and galanin.

These chemicals initiate sleep by sending a chemical chill pill to the arousal centres of the brain. Specialised brain cells called the orexin neurons, also located in the hypothalamus, help stabilise this process and keep you asleep.

Normal sleep goes through rhythmic sleep cycles, which usually repeat every 90 to 110 minutes. The cycles include alternating non-rapid eye movement (NREM) and rapid eye movement (REM) sleep. NREM sleep is further divided into stages of progressively deeper sleep. The higher the stage of NREM (stages progress from N1 to N3), the harder it is to wake someone. N1 is very light sleep, where you are drifting in and out of consciousness and are easily woken and, in my case, that tends to be when the light from Daniel's phone wakes me. For most people, the deepest sleep (N3) occurs more frequently in the first third of the night, while REM sleep predominates in the last third of the night.

You cycle through your sleep phases during the night and can re-enter N1 during brief arousal periods. N1 takes up about 2–5 per cent of your total sleep time, N2 accounts for 45–55 per cent of total sleep time and N3 sleep accounts for only 10–20 per cent of total sleep time.

REM sleep is named for the random rapid eye movements that occur during this phase. Your body is completely motionless, except for occasional muscle twitches, and big variations in heart rate, blood pressure and breathing rate. Experts say REM sleep is when dreaming happens. That's partly because of these rapid eye movements, but also because when people are woken up during REM sleep they often say they were dreaming – and frequently report they were vivid and bizarre dreams. REM sleep accounts for 20–25 per cent of your total sleep time; you go into REM sleep about four or five times in total in a typical night.

If you look at total sleep time, it decreases year on year until you hit about age 60, then it stays around the same after that. Ageing also sees you spending less time as a percentage in both either deep sleep or REM sleep compared to younger adults, and the time it takes to fall asleep increases slightly as well.

Why does your sleep go to the dogs as you age?

As you get older, a number of things happen to your brain to conspire against you sleeping well.

Many are indirect causes of lack of sleep. If you get hip or shoulder pain every time you roll over, your sleep will be worse. If your bladder (or prostate) or belly discomfort from reflux have you up and down all night, sleep will be broken. If your partner is a snorer, you can really struggle. All of these things are a part of getting older.

But it also seems that our brains are just less efficient at maintaining a decent slumber as we get older. But why?

Reduced brain rinsing

In Chapter 1, where I gave an overview of how the brain works, I discussed the glymphatic system, whereby fluid effectively rinses out the brain and removes the toxins that have snuck in by evading the blood–brain barrier or have been generated by metabolism in the brain cells themselves. This system is active during sleep.

Unfortunately, the glymphatic system degrades with age. So does our quality of sleep. Less sleep means less time to rinse the brain off and, as time goes by, the shower hose becomes faulty. This potentially means waste products can build up as sleep quality drops off.

The shrinking VLPO

Remember the ventrolateral preoptic area (or VLPO) in the brainstem which controls your sleep? This part of the brain sees a depletion in the number of cells as you age. Plus, it seems the connections within this part of the brain become more fragmented and don't work as seamlessly.

The circadian rhythm

The circadian rhythm is the 24-hour cycle of night and day that regulates our life, as it does for most living organisms. It is not just our sleep but our daily rhythms of physical activity and eating that also contribute to and are determined by our circadian rhythms.

This rhythm or internal body clock drives cyclical, predictable changes in our core body temperature (you cool down as you fall asleep), hormone changes (cortisol levels peak just before you wake up), heart rate, urine and gut function. Our circadian rhythm makes us sharpest during the day and helps us wind down and switch off at night.

This timing of the cycle is controlled by a kind of circadian pacemaker, the hypothalamic suprachiasmatic nucleus (SCN) in the base of the brain. It is sometimes called the body clock, using external cues such as sunlight, our activity levels and even our food intake. Influencing the innate circadian pacemaker is what scientists refer to as zeitgebers or external time cues.

Hormones that help your sleep

Sleep is so complex, with a range of drivers, but it turns out your brain comes pre-packaged with hormones that help this vital process happen seamlessly! Let's check them out.

Melatonin

Melatonin is a natural sleep hormone made by the pineal gland in the brain when the retinas at the back of your eyes stop receiving light signals. This melatonin directly hits the SCN and the first burst of melatonin releases after about two hours, which is followed by sleep. Your melatonin levels peak at 3 or 4 a.m. and then start to back off, which allows you to come naturally into lighter sleep and wake up without feeling groggy in the morning. Exactly *how* melatonin works its magic to send you off to sleep still isn't really understood.

Apart from its role in maintaining your body's own circadian rhythm or sleep–wake cycle, it's been proven to be a powerful anti-oxidant protecting the brain from damage. Natural melatonin levels increase from birth and peak around puberty but decline sharply in old age. This drop has been proposed as one of the primary reasons for the development of dementia.

Certainly, some studies suggest melatonin directly prevents the build-up of amyloid in the brain. And in other studies melatonin efficiently prevents that hyperphosphorylation of tau protein indirectly through its impact on enzymes that have been linked to brain cell degeneration (such as glycogen synthase kinase 3 beta (GSK3β) and cyclin-dependent kinase 5 (Cdk5). No wonder melatonin has been proposed as a potential medical treatment for Alzheimer's disease.

We still don't know for sure whether this *causes* circadian rhythm dysfunction or whether circadian dysfunction causes the melatonin levels to dwindle – which is why fixing your circadian rhythm is priority number one.

Orexin

Another key hormone in regulating sleep is orexin, which is sometimes called hypocretin. These peptide hormones contribute to keeping you awake by firing like crazy during the day but completely switching off when you're asleep. When they fire, they stimulate other neurons to release neurotransmitters that promote alertness, like noradrenaline, dopamine and serotonin. People with narcolepsy (where they constantly fall asleep) have between 85 and 90 per cent fewer orexin-producing neurons.

Recent studies have confirmed links between higher orexin levels and binge eating, pain, addiction and stress. Studies have shown that anxiety turbo charges your orexin levels, as does going into menopause, with a 300 per cent increase in orexin levels. This can be reversed with HRT. That doesn't guarantee you a brain that will be forever dementia-free, but maybe it can help a bit.

Cortisol

Cortisol is a hormone that is mainly released from your adrenal glands at times of stress. Its main role, when secreted in the Goldilocks amounts (i.e. the just right amount!) is to increase the body's metabolism of glucose, help control blood pressure and reduce inflammation. And, as we know, these are all critical for health.

Lots of health influencers have waged war on cortisol. That's because, while a bit is a boon for your body, prolonged high cortisol is a definite problem.

In response to stress, your body's first port of call is the sympathetic nervous system, which pumps out adrenaline. But if stress is prolonged, the brain tells the adrenals to release more cortisol to let the body continue to stay on high alert, mainly by releasing lots of sugar into the blood stream for ready use by the hungry brain. Consistently high levels of cortisol contribute not only to a lack of sleep but also weight gain, digestive issues, depression, anxiety, thinning skin and even diabetes.

Typically, the low point for cortisol levels is somewhere around midnight. Around two to three hours after you fall asleep they start to rise again, and keep rising into the waking hours, peaking at about 9 a.m. Then there is a slow decline during the course of the day.

But cortisol levels start to increase in the evening as we age and this increase is especially prominent in people over the age of 50, who struggle to sleep. It seems to affect REM sleep particularly.

Perimenopause is another time when your cortisol levels go up in general, but especially at night, and might be partly responsible for the crap sleep so many of us peri women experience. Good news: they tend to fall again after menopause proper.

Progesterone

Progesterone is the hormone released by your ovaries once you have ovulated. No ovulation = no progesterone. One of progesterone's many roles is that it has sedative properties. So even young women with natural cycles tend to have more disrupted sleep before their period starts, when progesterone levels have fallen to their lowest point. But in perimenopause, even well before the hot flushes have started, most of us will get sporadic ovulation and encounter progesterone-free cycles for the first time. Without that sedative on board, it's no wonder that perimenopause is a time when sleep can be most elusive.

Why sleep is critical for brain health

As we know, we used to think sleep was just a passive thing your brain did when there was nothing much else going on, so it just shut down. Well, that entire concept has been turned on its head.

At a cellular level, sleep is critical for the elimination of waste and restoration of depleted energy sources inside the brain, as well as neuroplasticity (although we're not 100 per cent sure *how* this happens). Sleep is the time when we consolidate our memories. But not *all* memories. Somehow our brain knows to give preference to those specific memories that will be important to us in the future. Think learning, facts or emotionally important events.

Sleep also affects many other brain functions. Sleep deprivation impairs performance on tasks that test cognitive ability, short-term memory and acting impulsively in response to stress.

Studies in mice models shows that sleep helps the maintenance cells in our brain to start housekeeping of the most heavily used synapses. Repeated or chronic sleep deprivation activates the microglia, which can lead to a state of sustained microglia over-activation, perhaps increasing the brain's susceptibility to damage.

Beyond the brain, sleep kickstarts the immune system. But in a healthy way. After just one bad night's sleep, nerve fibres from your sympathetic nervous system release the neurotransmitter noradrenaline into the blood stream. This chemical stimulates the adrenal glands to release adrenaline into the blood stream. It also kickstarts a range of pro-inflammatory chemicals. Generalised inflammation, as we know, has a whole raft of negative effects, including on your brain.

What is the connection between sleep and dementia?

Sleep disturbance is a *symptom* of dementia. Studies have shown that around 70 per cent of people with diagnosed cognitive impairment or dementia have some sort of sleep disturbances. And this is linked to a poorer prognosis. But maybe the sleep disturbance is just a quasi-biomarker for dementia severity, rather than the cause?

Professor Sharon Naismith is the Chair of Psychology at the Charles Perkins Centre, the University of Sydney and also heads up the Healthy Brain Ageing Program at the Brain and Mind Centre. She has examined the interplay between sleep and ageing. Much of the evidence on the association between sleep duration and dementia comes from studies with a follow-up of less than 10 years, she explained. As most dementias take 20 years or more to declare themselves, until recently it's been hard to prove the cause-and-effect relationship. In addition, 'many of the studies haven't controlled for obstructive sleep apnoea or depression,' she points out.

But the data is starting to emerge. I already mentioned the 2017 meta-analysis of 27 studies covering almost 70,000 people that found that sleep problems raise the risk of cognitive impairment by 65 per cent, and that poor quality sleep could explain as many as 15 per cent of cases of Alzheimer's disease. However, those studies did have some methodological flaws.

But researchers are excited about the Whitehall Studies, which are large long-term studies of almost 30,000 civil servants between the ages of 20 and 64, who have been followed up on a whole raft of metrics since 1967. And they are still ongoing. Because the follow-up is so long, their data is super interesting.

From a Whitehall study published in 2021, we now know that persistent short sleep duration at age 50, 60 and 70 was linked to a 30 per cent increased dementia risk, independent of a whole bunch of other risk factors.

> The current thinking is that the relationship between lack of sleep is bidirectional. This means that the brain changes that underpin dementia can disrupt sleep, and sleep disturbance contributes to the development of dementia. So when you get both sleep disturbances and dementia at the same time, you get a more rapid decline. But the biggest takeaway is that while there is some chicken *and* egg, the jury is now *in*: getting your sleep sorted in midlife is critical for protecting your brain!

But before we leave this, it is important to know that this is not a case of 'more is more'. Professor Naismith points to a U-shaped curve in which people who either sleep the longest or the shortest have the highest risk of developing dementia. One study of almost 28,000 people in China and the UK, reported in 2020, found that more than 10 hours of sleep a day upped the risk as much as having less than four hours a day.

'Six to eight hours a day seems to be the sweet spot,' Professor Naismith told me. 'And napping counts.' (More on that later.)

What the experts do to maintain brain health
PROFESSOR SHARON NAISMITH

Sharon prioritises her sleep and does what she can to improve it. She rides a bicycle three to four times a week and does weights and cardio training. As a busy mum she was always putting herself last but has started to try and shift the balance a bit. 'I'm trying to bring hobbies back into my life.'

In terms of diet, she has tried in the past to aim for calorie restriction. 'But I'm not disciplined enough to do those diets.' She isn't too hard on herself, staying as healthy as she can while trying not to obsess over it. As a former barista and cafe owner, she sees enormous value in coffee beyond the health benefits and has two to three a day.

Quantity vs quality sleep?

It's not just quantity of sleep that counts. Quality matters. There was a small Korean study published in 2018 that only followed people up for four years. The researchers found that those who struggled to fall asleep had double the risk of cognitive decline over the four-year period than people who hit the pillow and went out like a light, even when total time spent asleep was fine. It's possible that trouble falling asleep is an early warning signal that something is afoot in the brain.

A 2016 German study of 800 people found that those with broken sleep were more likely to go on to develop cognitive decline after three years. But those who struggled to get to sleep were okay – as long as once they fell asleep their sleep was good quality.

Most experts agree that sleep quality, not just sleep duration, is important for reducing your dementia risk.

How do we know whether you're a good or bad sleeper?

Typically, we analyse sleep formally through polysomnography, which is also known as a sleep study. These can be done in a sleep clinic or at home. The scientist measures your eye movements, brain and muscle activity, breathing, blood oxygen levels, body positioning and movements, snoring, and heart rate while you sleep.

But even if you don't have access to a sleep study, you probably have a pretty good idea about your own sleep quality. 'By and large if someone says they're a bad sleeper, they are,' Professor Sharon Naismith told me.

Could there be other things going on to disrupt your sleep?

Aches and pains from a raft of joint and muscle issues can disrupt sleep, as can hot flushes, running to the toilet and depression, which stuffs up sleep all by itself. I'll deal with these soon.

Is insomnia genetic?

Yep! If you come from a family of bad sleepers, sorry! Studies suggest that between 30 and 40 per cent of insomnia is in your genes (up to 250 of them have been identified so far). We even know which genes (although you can't get the gene tests yet unless you're part of a study). They all affect different neurotransmitters.

Even if you are a genetic poor sleeper, we don't have special treatments for you yet and you have to muck in and do all the other things we will chat about in this chapter to wrangle your nights back into line.

However, if you're not waking feeling refreshed and someone in your house is moaning about your snoring, there might be something else going on.

Sleep disordered breathing and sleep apnoea

Sleep disordered breathing, or SDB, encompasses a group of conditions where there is some kind of abnormal respiratory pattern during sleep. The most common is sleep apnoea, also known as obstructive sleep apnoea, which happens when your throat is partly or completely blocked while you are asleep, causing you to stop breathing intermittently through the night.

These apnoeas, or periods of no breathing, can last anywhere between 10 and 90 seconds, after which you will usually wake briefly (although you might not remember waking up the next morning). Apnoeas can happen multiple times a night. Doctors grade the condition from mild to severe depending on the number of times it happens, how long the apnoeas last and how much your blood oxygen levels fall when it does happen.

Sleep apnoea gets more common the older you are and also the heavier you are, as a big jaw and neck can increase the chance of your throat blocking off. There is also often a family history of sleep apnoea.

You might not know you have it. But here are some signs to look out for:

- stopping breathing while sleeping, which is more likely to be noticed by your partner or someone in the next room when you go away!
- snoring

- tossing and turning
- waking up feeling like you are choking
- waking up feeling tired and unrefreshed after sleep
- headaches.

Why does this all matter? Because while sleep disordered breathing affects 30 per cent of adults overall, it can affect up to 60 per cent of older adults, especially men. But it affects 70 to 80 per cent of people with dementia, and the severity of the sleep apnoea increases with dementia severity. Does that mean sleep disordered breathing increases your risk of cognitive decline and dementia? It certainly looks that way. Professor Naismith says that having sleep apnoea increases your risk of dementia by 26 per cent.

Many experts assert that there is probably a 'bidirectional link' between disturbed sleep and dementia so that you end up with a positive-feedback loop in which dementia-type illnesses exacerbate SDB, and vice versa.

Fixing your sleep!

There are quite a few things that can be tried to fix your sleep and I have covered them here, in the order you should try them.

STEP 1: CIRCADIAN RHYTHM REPAIR

Professor Ian Hickie has done an enormous amount of research into improving circadian rhythms, and as far as he is concerned, in 100 per cent of cases, this is the place to start. 'Morning sunlight and physical activity are the biggest drivers of circadian rhythms,' he said.

We know from research that the later you get your face into the sunshine to switch off your melatonin that is produced at night, the harder you will find it to get to sleep at a decent hour. If you are someone who struggles to regulate your body clock, five minutes spent outdoors on a balcony in the morning sun will do you the world of good.

Early morning exposure to sunlight switches off your main sleep hormone, melatonin. But for this shutdown to happen you need a light intensity of at least 1500 lux (brighter than standard artificial lighting). I ask my patients who are struggling with their sleep to have their morning cup of tea or coffee outside in the sunlight, even in the rain (grab an umbrella) to use natural light as a powerful zeitgeber (or natural regulator).

At the other end of the day, being in bright light will delay the revving up of your melatonin levels and delay your natural circadian rhythm. So dim the lights about an hour before you want to go to sleep.

PHYSICAL ACTIVITY

I'll talk about the strong link between exercise and good sleep soon but exercise can be used as a zeitgeber to enhance your sleep if you exercise at a regular time every day.

Obtaining study evidence that links exercise with less insomnia has been a bit fraught. In 2017, a meta-analysis of five trials of structured exercise programs for mid-life women with insomnia found that there were minimal, statistically insignificant benefits for insomnia. Within that meta-analysis, rigorous exercise like aerobics improved sleep more than exercise with low levels of physical activity (like yoga).

In a 2021 study from Hong Kong of older adults with an average age of 67, both a 12-week program of brisk walking and strength training exercises and a 12-week Tai Chi program improved sleep. And these benefits were still going at the end of the two-year study.

GET INTO A DECENT ROUTINE

We saw sleep go to custard for many of us in the pandemic as nobody left their homes, evening drinks eventually started at 10 a.m., sleep happened whenever, and meals, bedtime, work hours and showers were random. That link between a lack of routine and bad sleep is well known.

Ian Hickie suspects one of the reasons staying in the workforce keeps you young is the routine that it brings with it. Retiring on a beach will see most people lose all structure in their day and develop both worse sleep and cognitive function.

But we can fix this. An interesting Israeli study showed that people who followed a regular daily routine (not just bed time and morning sunshine but regular meals, exercising and even showering) fell asleep more quickly and improved their sleep quality and quantity.

STEP 2: SLEEP HYGIENE FOR SLEEP REPAIR

Bad sleepers often have developed bad habits over years or even decades that seem to program their brains not to sleep. The idea of sleep hygiene is to clean up your bad sleep habits and retrain your brain to know when it's sleep time and when it's not. Strong sleep hygiene incorporates all the circadian rhythm stuff *plus* having a bedroom environment that helps you to sleep. Sure, we're talking a decent mattress, a good fan and blinds. But keeping a stable sleep schedule and following a relaxing pre-bed routine also contribute to great sleep hygiene.

Here are the most important sleep hygiene steps to take to rewire your brain:

- **Wind down.** You need a wind-down period before bed to help your brain stop becoming stimulated. This usually takes a good hour or so. No screens of any kind, TV, iPad, iPhone, etc. Also no heart-stopping books or arguments! Instead, try soft music, an aromatherapy bath, dim lights, and maybe a nice orgasm if you have a partner who is willing and able!
- **Your bed is for sex and sleep only.** There is a fallacy that 'just resting' in bed is good for your brain. But it actually has the opposite effect, making it harder for your brain to fall asleep later

on and wrecking your sleep hygiene! No phones, no Facebook, no Netflix, no Instagram in bed.

- **Relax.** Once you get into bed (or have finished having sex), practise progressive muscular relaxation in which you relax your muscles one by one from the tips of your toes to the top of your head. There is some evidence for yoga, abdominal breathing and progressive muscle relaxation too.

- **The 15-minute rule.** Give yourself 15 minutes to fall asleep. If your mind starts to wander or you feel tense, get up and leave the room for a short time, somewhere between 10 and 30 minutes, and then return to bed as if you were starting the night again. It doesn't matter what you do as long as you don't overstimulate your brain with a screen. You can even get some ironing done. If you're awake anyway, at least you'll achieve some productive work and not feel quite as frustrated as you would when you're just lying and watching the clock for hours at a time.

STEP 3: COGNITIVE BEHAVIOURAL THERAPY FOR INSOMNIA (CBT-I)

This technique is designed to stamp out annoying middle-of-the-night awakenings. The cornerstone is actually *restricting* sleep. That starts with restricting the time spent in bed. Then you progress to gradually increasing the time spent in bed. The initial time in bed is usually the average nightly total sleep time over the last week. However, the time allowed in bed should not be less than 5.5 hours, even for people who sleep less than 5.5 hours per night.

For example, consider a person who goes to bed at 11 p.m. and gets out of bed at 8 a.m. but sleeps on average only six hours per night. During the first step of this procedure this person will be in bed only six hours (e.g. 12 a.m. to 6 a.m.). This sounds harsh but after a week or so there will be a marked decrease in time spent awake in the middle of the night.

In 2019, a meta-analysis of 13 trials found that people receiving just four–six sessions of cognitive behavioural therapy for insomnia (CBT-I) reported their sleep really improved. These improvements were generally well maintained for three to 12 months post-treatment.

STEP 4: HERBAL AND 'NATURAL' OPTIONS

If none of the above works, you might want to head to a health food store or the natural remedies section of your local pharmacy. The range of effective herbal and natural supplements that target sleep is wide, and I don't want to leave any of them out. So, mosey your way through this long list below.

St John's wort (*Hypericum perforatum*) Mostly studied as an anti-anxiety and antidepressant supplement, there is also a *little* bit of evidence for St John's wort improving sleep as well. There have been numerous small studies, involving 10 volunteers at a time, but they haven't shown any significant benefits yet. So taking it in the evening in the hope that you'll have a nice long, sound sleep is pointless. But if you are taking it for anxiety or depression relief, and it works, you might see your sleep improve.

The standard dose is 300 mg three times a day with meals. If you use it properly it's very safe, and apart from some minor tummy upset and your skin becoming more sensitive to sunlight (so burning more easily), there are few nasty side effects. It interacts with so many medications, including the Pill, antidepressants and antihistamines, that I'd urge you just to run it by your pharmacist first.

5-hydroxy-tryptophan This amino acid, commonly found in dairy foods, is the immediate precursor of serotonin. It is thought to act by increasing the synthesis of serotonin. When you have natural tryptophan as part of your diet, you're also eating a stack of other large amino acids that compete for the system that transports them all into the brain. So it doesn't actually raise your brain tryptophan levels. A bedtime glass of milk or cheese sandwich as promoted by some TikTok influencers will be useless for people with insomnia.

But it can be purchased as an over-the-counter dietary supplement in some countries. Tryptophan, at a dose of 1 g taken 45 minutes before bedtime, will see you fall asleep more quickly if you have mild insomnia, especially if you usually take ages to fall asleep. At this dose, it has no effect on sleep architecture, and won't leave you drowsy the next day. The data is less compelling for its ability to give you a longer or higher quality sleep. Also, if you have moderate or severe insomnia, tryptophan is less effective. Although the effect of tryptophan on sleep has been studied only over the short term, researchers believe that its effect is not likely to change, given that a 1-g dose taken at bedtime will be completely metabolised before the end of the night.

Ashwagandha (*Withania somnifera*) This plant has been touted in India as a treatment for everything from arthritis to attention deficit hyperactivity disorder, insomnia to tuberculosis, asthma to backache, Parkinson's disease to an under-active thyroid.

A 2021 meta-analysis of five studies (all conducted in India and with one company sponsor) of ashwagandha for insomnia was positive. All five trials found a significant improvement in overall sleep in the ashwagandha extract compared to placebo. Three of the trials looked at mental alertness the next morning, and all three were better for ashwagandha than placebo. Ditto anxiety levels in the three trials that asked about this. There were few side effects.

On the downside the trials were small and all used different doses. But the authors concluded that ashwagandha at doses at or over 600 mg/day and taken for eight weeks or more is the most effective way to go.

STEP 5: MEDICATIONS FOR BETTER SLEEP

Studies show that around 40 per cent of adults with insomnia have used either over-the-counter medication or alcohol to help induce sleep, and approximately one-quarter have used prescription medications at least once.

They're never the best place to start and should be a last resort. But sleep deprivation is a torture chamber and I wouldn't tell my patients who are at the end of their tether and risking their brain health to suck it up. There are times when these are necessary. They're best for short-term, targeted treatment while you get your circadian rhythms, your sleep hygiene and everything sorted out!

Melatonin supplements There is evidence that taking a melatonin supplement can help with poor sleep.

In terms of dose, most of the data comes out in front for 2 mg at night. However, many people use much higher doses. Certainly, many of my patients tell me they sleep better with 5 mg melatonin than 2 mg. Even higher doses are available. The data we have suggests that higher doses are safe, even doses above 10 mg. The worry is that higher doses might cause desensitisation of melatonin receptors so that over time, it stops working as effectively.

Orexin receptor antagonists As you know, the orexins are peptides produced by neurons of the lateral hypothalamus that are responsible for keeping you awake. In an ideal world they should be completely dormant during your sleep.

We now have ways to switch them off at night-time by using prescription medications that sit on their receptors in the brain and switch them off, not on. These orexin receptor antagonists have been shown to improve sleep quality and sleep architecture in people with insomnia with very few side effects (although a bit of drowsiness the next day can happen).

MEDICATIONS WITH SLEEPINESS AS A SIDE EFFECT

Your doctor might try to help you with medications that aren't designed to battle insomnia but their side effects make you drowsy and might be used occasionally off-label for this purpose.

Antihistamines Diphenhydramine and doxylamine are over-the-counter 'first-generation' antihistamines that have sedation as a side effect. They're also the main ingredient in a lot of the over-the-counter sleeping tablets you can get at the pharmacy. They last in your body for around nine hours so many people feel a bit like they are hungover the next morning. In my experience they work well for an occasional night of sleep, with no addiction. Best for Friday nights or a time when an antihistamine hangover won't ruin your day!!

Diphenhydramine is not recommended for the elderly as it can cause falls and confusion.

Antidepressants at low dose Popular antidepressants with good sleep effects include mirtazapine, amitriptyline and agomelatine, which probably help you sleep through their action on your brain's serotonin levels. They have best evidence when there is insomnia and depression.

Benzodiazepine sleeping pills These are your classic 'tran-quillisers'. They work by activating the GABA receptors in the brain, mimicking the GABA relaxation and sleep-inducing properties. The big issue with these sleeping pills is addiction and rebound insomnia when you stop using them. I do prescribe them for short-term use for insomnia during a crisis. For example, I have prescribed them for patients who lost a job or found out their partner has cancer and literally could not sleep a wink. But they can only be used for a maximum of two weeks before you start running into issues.

COMPLEMENTARY AND ALTERNATIVE MEDICINES FOR SLEEP

Before we start looking at these medications, I just want to say a quick word about the placebo effect. One 2020 study set out to look at the placebo effect in trials for products to combat insomnia. The study recruited 117 volunteers with sleep difficulties. Only some of the volunteers received a proven treatment. However, all the people in the study reported lower insomnia severity, less fatigue and a higher perception of sleep quality, confirming the placebo effect is brilliant for insomnia. Therefore, everything I'm about to say comes with the caveat of maybe it's a placebo effect.

Omega-3s Epidemiological studies have linked eating more fish with better sleep. Could it be the omega-3s which are high in fish? Animal studies suggest that docosahexaenoic acid (DHA), one of the key active components of omega-3 oils, helps with regulating your brain's natural melatonin production.

A randomised controlled trial in 2021 showed that 1 g of an omega-3 supplement twice daily (each containing 180 mg EPA and 120 mg DHA) improved insomnia in women who were being treated with hormone blockers for breast cancer and were therefore in a chemical menopause. After just four weeks of treatment, the women who took omega-3 reported better sleep, less depression, and better mood than those who took a placebo. But it didn't happen that night.

Omega-3s are very well tolerated, with few side effects. Some studies have linked omega-3 supplements with prostate cancer, but the jury is out on whether there's anything to worry about. If you're taking medicine that affects blood clotting or if you're allergic to fish or shellfish, check in with your doctor or pharmacist first before taking them.

Chamomile In 2011, we got the results of a randomised, double-blind, placebo-controlled trial of 34 insomniacs. Patients either took

270 mg chamomile twice daily or a placebo for 28 days. Unfortunately, the people taking the chamomile didn't have any better sleep than those on the placebo. Then again, it was very well tolerated. I found some chamomile supplements online and they were pretty cheap!

Vitamin B6 We have plenty of anecdotal evidence that indicates vitamin B6 (pyridoxine) supplements taken before bed enhance the vividness of your dreams, as well as your ability to remember the dreams the next day. A small 2002 pilot study seemed to confirm this and the authors reported that the higher the dose of the vitamin B6 the higher the people in the study rated the vividness, bizarreness and colour of their dreams. A subsequent Australian study found that vitamin B6 certainly increased the ability to remember dreams, while a B complex vitamin pill before bed made sleep quality worse overall. Hmmmm. I don't like the sound of that at all! So possibly B6 is it.

Magnesium supplements Magnesium is a mineral found in fibre-rich foods. Think dark green veggies, like kale, along with legumes such as kidney beans, nuts and whole grains, and also dairy foods. In blood tests on my patients, magnesium deficiency is super common. Small studies have found that magnesium supplements may help people fall asleep quicker, sleep longer overall and boost melatonin levels. It also seems to help people with restless leg syndrome. It might be because it appears to increase the amount of the neurotransmitter GABA in the brain. This can effectively slow your head down, allowing your brain to switch off and fall asleep. You can't overdose on magnesium in foods, but you can take too many supplements, especially if they're bound to a chemical that can upset your guts. Forms of magnesium, like magnesium carbonate, chloride and oxide, can all cause stomach cramps and diarrhoea. It's better to use magnesium glycinate or magnesium gluconate.

Passionflower *Passiflora incarnata* (Purple passionflower) is an indigenous American vine with white and purple flowers and an edible fruit. In tiny clinical trials *Passiflora* extracts showed anti-anxiety effects, including as a pre-med before surgery. And in mice it's a great sedative. The human data is a bit thin on the ground. Having said that, it appears to be pretty safe, so not much downside other than stress on your wallet.

Lemon balm I see so many peri and menopausal patients, I feel like I talk about insomnia multiple times a day. So, when a few of my patients touted a supplement by an online brand that got rid of their insomnia altogether, I was intrigued. It turns out the main ingredient was lemon balm, AKA *Melissa officinalis* L., leaf extract.

An Italian study gave a commercial preparation of lemon balm to 20 stressed-out volunteers. The volunteers took the supplement twice a day for 15 days and they did report a 42 per cent reduction in insomnia. But with no placebo control and a company-sponsored trial, I'm sceptical. I bought a bottle of one of these supplements online to give them a whirl. It cost me $36 for a bottle of 60 tablets, which the pack says should last me a month as I should take two at night only. I think I have tried it on 20 different nights, and it doesn't do anything for me. But I didn't follow the trial rules, I didn't do it for 15 days in a row.

I think there is better out there.

Valerian root Derived from the *Valeriana officinalis* plant, valerian attaches to both the GABA and serotonin receptors in the brain and makes you sleepier and a bit cheerier. In 2015, a meta-analysis of studies of valerian was published. From those trials you could say there is some evidence of improvement in sleep with valerian if you take it for two weeks or more, at least on subjective testing. But the studies were of poor quality and the authors weren't keen to make firm recommendations.

I am going to 'fess up that this is my go-to supplement for sleep. Maybe it's the placebo effect, but it works a treat for me. The one I take is from the supermarket and costs $28 for 60 tablets. It is meant to last 30 to 60 days because the instruction is to take one to two tablets at night. I only need one. It has some other ingredients including magnesium, licorice, hops, China root (*Wolfiporia cocos*) and *Anemarrhena asphodeloides* extract, so saying it is the valerian that is responsible is a bit tricky.

Aromatherapy This is where you gently inhale various essential oils with the aim of the scents having calming and hypnotic effects on the brain. It can be practised in a few ways. The oil can be directly applied to your skin. That's going to be pretty strong, so it can be diluted with a carrier oil such as sweet almond oil. You can dab the oil onto your temples, forehead and wrists before bedtime. Or you could apply a few drops of essential oil onto a cottonwool ball and slip it inside your pillowcase at night. Or you could try having a bath with a few drops of essential oil added to the water. Some people add essential oil drops to a humidifier or vaporiser in the bedroom at bedtime or add a few drops of essential oil to a warm damp cloth and put this over their forehead or neck.

The evidence for essential oils for insomnia tends to come from small trials, but in 2021, a meta-analysis of 34 studies showed that aromatherapy was highly effective in improving sleep problems such as insomnia and poor sleep quality. The best evidence in this analysis was seen with lavender. But other trials have shown some benefits from using essential oils of chamomile, ylang ylang, jasmine, bergamot and sweet marjoram.

Some people have very sensitive skin and can get rashes if they come in direct contact with some essential oils. So, test a very small amount on your skin first.

Acupressure In a randomised controlled trial of 50 residents in aged care facilities, five weeks of standard acupressure on the HT7 (Shenmen) points of both wrists significantly reduced insomnia, and kept the residents sleeping soundly two weeks after the trial ended. Not much downside!

Cannabis CBD Let's go through some definitions first. The plant *cannabis sativa* is the one we recognise, with its longish green leaves. It contains more than 80 different chemicals known as cannabinoids. The most abundant cannabinoid, tetrahydrocannabinol (THC), is well known for its psychoactive properties (it makes you feel stoned), while cannabidiol (CBD) is the second-most abundant cannabinoid and it is non-psychoactive.

Cannabis plants and derivatives that have less than 0.3 per cent THC are classified as 'hemp'. In many countries, hemp is no longer defined as a controlled substance by the government. Many hemp products are marketed as CBD products.

Once a confirmed 'alternative therapy', these days a growing number of people are getting it on a prescription from their doctor. So where is the evidence? In short, it's in its infancy.

In a 2020 study of older adults with chronic pain, people using medicinal cannabis slept better throughout the night. But the authors noticed that people got used to the cannabis if they used it frequently and it became less effective over time. Separately, a 2020 meta-analysis of five studies (two randomised controlled trials and three non-randomised studies) with a total of 219 study participants was published. The authors couldn't conclude anything. The differences in the studies, their participants, the doses, the possible bias and their wildly differing results all meant a big shoulder shrug for insomnia. A 2022 paper suggested that i) because studies have been inconclusive for effectiveness, ii) that cannabis can interact with medications including antidepressants, making them less effective, and iii) the fact that cannabis products can cause daytime sleepiness and impair driving capacity, people with insomnia should look elsewhere for support.

I do refer my patients who want to try cannabis oil to doctors who prescribe it. Some have great results. Some don't. It is very expensive but I think if that's what you want to do, give it a shot.

Other sleep hacks

I have spent years chatting to patients and experts, and experimenting on friends and family trying to come up with a range of other steps that you might not have thought of to help get more sleep. Not all will work for everyone, but many are worth at least a try!

COOL IT!

Maximum sleepiness occurs when your core body temperature is at its lowest. So feeling overheated can be a real killer for your sleep.

Anyone who hears me talk about menopause is sick of me saying you *do not need to put up with* hot flushes or night sweats. But now that you know that the hot flushes that are wrecking your sleep are also damaging your brain, it's time to get pro-active about this.

Which leads me to fixing your hot flushes if you have them. There are *so many* treatments for hot flushes and night sweats from menopause. And yes, hormone replacement therapy is a super good option for many women. Nobody can sleep through hot flushes so go see your GP for some help.

BLADDER RENOVATION

If you are someone who would have a reasonable sleep but for the regular night-time trips to the toilet, help is at hand! It is part of a spectrum of symptoms that come with an overactive bladder associated with ageing (not from having a baby). Your GP can give you advice but my tips include getting off caffeine (check if that helps), switching from fizzy drinks, including soda water, to still, and making sure you are not feeling constipated. And while there's nothing wrong with doing pelvic floor exercises, they won't help with the night-time trots to the loo. But there are medications that do help. Just be careful as these medications can cause confusion in the elderly. But for people in midlife, they tend to have few side effects.

FIX YOUR ACHES AND PAINS

As a GP I see lots of people with chronic (ongoing) aches and pains from various causes and this often interferes with sleep. While not all aches and pains are fixable, I would at least see your GP about simple interventions, like a short-term anti-inflammatory medication or a steroid injection into hip or shoulder bursitis, or a referral to physiotherapy for some pain relief.

Chronic pain is a complex beast and we are learning more about it all the time. There is a feeling among my patients that pain X must be caused directly by injury X and to fix pain X the only options are diagnosing and treating injury X or taking strong painkillers or both. We now know that pain and the original injury usually correlate poorly. I often see people with scans so horrific I can't believe they're walking around, only to be told they have almost no pain. I have more patients who have the opposite situation. They are debilitated by their chronic pain and are utterly frustrated that despite experiencing what they describe as agony, only a minor problem is found on a scan. That's because chronic pain is complex and your wellbeing, your emotional health and the way your nerves are wired all contribute to your experience of the pain.

If we can't fix the original injury (because it's minor and is not appropriate for surgery or because all the interventions we do don't work), we are faced with a choice between strong painkillers that are choc-full of side effects, including cognitive impairments, addiction and horrid constipation, and alternatives.

I don't have space here to talk too much about this but we know from studies that non-painkiller options work. These include regular exercise (often at least initially supervised by an exercise physiologist to make sure you are doing them the right way). In addition, we can use heat packs, yoga and Tai Chi, music therapy, biofeedback, therapeutic massage and mind–body techniques, often delivered by a counsellor.

A quick note about aches and pains in menopause. Studies show musculoskeletal symptoms can hit up to 80 per cent of women going through menopause. In some studies, these symptoms are more common than hot flushes, especially among Asian women.

Different studies have yielded different results but there is some evidence that hormone replacement therapy can help.

COMBAT REFLUX

That heartburn feeling can come on at night when your horizontal position allows food from your stomach to easily flow back up into your windpipe and burn! That's especially true if you had a late dinner which hasn't emptied out of your stomach when you hit the sack. Try eating dinner earlier, tilting the head of your bed up slightly (you can fold a towel or two and put it under the head of your mattress or put a couple of bricks under the feet at the head of the bed). If that doesn't work, see your doctor about whether you need some tests to diagnose the condition properly and get some treatment.

CUT BACK EXCESS ALCOHOL

Alcohol makes lots of people drowsy. But that doesn't mean alcohol helps you sleep well. Quite the opposite. It stuffs up the quality of your sleep. Specifically, it blocks REM sleep, which is your restorative sleep.

There are a few reasons for this. The volume of liquid can make you need to pee through the night, it can make oesophageal reflux worse, which can cause heartburn, and it can make sleep disordered breathing or sleep apnoea worse. Stick to one to two drinks a night for better sleep.

What about napping?

For the purposes of this chapter I am going to define napping as 'a short sleep, typically taken during daylight hours'. Scientists break down napping into three types:

- the prophylactic nap: a nap taken in anticipation of sleep loss
- the replacement nap: a nap taken in response to sleep loss
- the appetitive nap: a nap taken for convenience and/or enjoyment.

In terms of protecting the brain, it seems to be all about the length of the nap. Studies coalesce around benefits with a clearly defined one-hour cut-off. Naps of over an hour have been linked to everything from higher risks of Parkinson's disease to heart disease to higher all-cause mortality (death from any cause). Long nappers are also more likely to be obese and have symptoms that suggest they suffer from depression. On the flip side, shorter naps of less than an hour have been found to be mildly protective.

In terms of brain health, we see a pretty similar pattern emerging. Naps of over an hour increase the risk of cognitive decline over time. Naps under an hour seem to be less harmful and possibly beneficial. One Japanese study found that napping for less than 30 minutes (power napping) halved the risk of cognitive impairment over a five-year period. That reflects similar data that shows that taking a nap for less than 30 minutes actually turbo charges brain performance plus your ability to learn new facts. But wait! There's more! Another 2011 study found that taking a nap (length of time didn't matter) blocked and even reversed feelings of anger and fear and made people rate themselves as happier. The trick with this study was that you have to enter REM sleep during your nap to get the benefits.

What nobody has been able to clarify is the chicken-and-egg situation: do people who are a bit less healthy in general feel the need to take a nap? So is the nap a biomarker for being unwell? Or is the napping the cause of the reduced brain function? Some studies have found that napping beyond an hour interferes with your night-time sleep and that could impact on your health.

I have tried to be a power napper and am an abysmal failure at it. If I can fall asleep during the day I wake up feeling like someone has hit me over the head. All power to those who can. But if you're going to nap, set your alarm clock to stop you from sleeping more than an hour. If you can master this, it may well be a boon for your brain.

I feel that sleep is so crucial to every aspect of life. Whether we're talking about teen mental health, menopause symptoms, weight loss or preventing dementia, this topic is central. It is worth the effort to get it right.

Takeaways

- Most experts agree that sleep quality, not just sleep duration, is important for reducing your dementia risk.
- Having more sleep (greater than 10 hours) is just as bad as having minimal sleep (four or less hours). Six to eight hours a night is optimal.
- Having a sleep disorder like sleep apnoea can significantly increase the risk of developing dementia, especially for men.
- Creating a great sleep hygiene routine is crucial to improving broken sleep. Look at fixing your circadian rhythm, increasing exposure to morning sunlight, regular physical activity, and a set routine to wind down before bed.
- Napping is okay as long as it does not go over 30 minutes during the day, as this can affect night-time sleep. A nap of less than 30 minutes can help increase cognition . . . which is why it has been labelled the power nap!

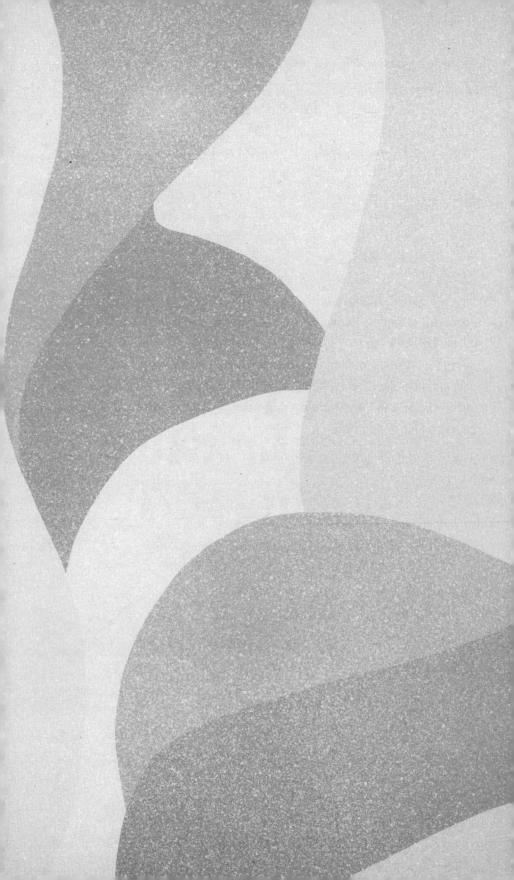

CHAPTER 10

Why does dementia affect women more than men?

My absolute passion is women's health and menopause, and the transition into menopause or perimenopause in particular. So, no book I ever write would be complete without a deep dive into the impact of hormones, especially as there seems to be such a correlation between the female primary sex hormones and the development of dementia.

Dementia is the biggest killer of women in Australia, where I live. Two out of every three people with dementia are women. Women are 55 per cent more likely to get dementia than men, and once they hit mild cognitive impairment, women progress more quickly to dementia than men. Brain scans tell us that the rate at which brain cells are dying in the brain is faster in women than in men. Why?

Professor Rebecca Thurston, Professor of Psychiatry, Psychology and Epidemiology at the University of Pittsburgh, has led much of the research into the relationship between gender, menopause, and brain and cardiovascular health. 'I don't think we know for sure,' she told me.

One possibility she points out is that women live longer than men, which gives them more opportunity to get dementia. Some studies have found that men and women have the same rate of dementia up to age 80, at which point rates in women race ahead. And given that women live longer than men, this age cut-off could be to blame.

But maybe there are other things going on? A recent study found that around the world, women's reduced access to education could be at play here. But even that doesn't seem to be the full story. 'There is data that women do have a higher susceptibility to dementia,' Professor Thurston says.

Hormones and the brain

The female primary sex hormone oestrogen totally affects the brain. Women don't just get more dementia than men: they also get more migraines, anxiety and depression. Now let's unpick *why* and what you can do about it!

How does oestrogen affect the brain?

Oestrogen seems to protect your brain. One 2019 study in the journal *Neurology* reported on almost 16,000 women who were followed from 1964 to 2017. Forty-two per cent of the women developed dementia. Women who went through a natural menopause at age 47.4 (which in this study was the mean menopause age) or younger had a 19 per cent higher dementia risk than women who went through menopause later. Shorter reproductive spans (i.e. the years between when a female gets her first period and menopause) of less than 34.4 years (which again was the mean duration in this study) were associated with 20 per cent higher dementia risk.

Your brain (regardless of your gender) is riddled with oestrogen receptors. They're everywhere, but your prefrontal cortex and hippocampus have a particularly high density of oestrogen. Oestrogen helps repair and maintain neurons, plus reduces inflammation, cell death (known as apoptosis) and tau hyperphosphorylation (which is, as we know, a key hallmark of neuron damage in Alzheimer's disease).

Animal studies indicate that oestrogen influences the organisation of the neurons and their synapses within the hippocampus and prefrontal cortex, which are parts of the brain that are essential for memory coding. It also seems to be an actual neurotransmitter.

Specifically, the most significant effect of oestrogen on cognitive function is probably on verbal memory, which is a broad term for memories that come from what you read or hear.

Progesterone

Progesterone is produced by the ovaries during the second half of the menstrual cycle. It plays an important role in a normal menstrual cycle and is essential for maintaining the early stages of pregnancy. But what does this have to do with the brain?

Progesterone has a significant protective effect in the brain. It promotes new nerve growth, repairs myelin, reduces inflammation and 'reactive gliosis', which is the effect of the brain reacting to injury or trauma. It pumps up the number of brain immune cells which rush to the injured area and start healing the damaged tissue.

What do perimenopause and menopause do to the brain?

Menopause hits officially one year from your last period. That's it. It is a single day that you often only identify in retrospect. Everything after that day is your post-menopause. And leading up to menopause is your menopause transition, also known as perimenopause. This phase lasts between 4.37 and 8.57 years and it's the phase I call hormone hell. During this phase up to 80 per cent of women get hot flushes, 25 per cent have mega-heavy periods, and about 10 per cent experience sore boobs. And your brain is affected possibly most brutally of all, with symptoms such as mood swings and brain fog, two of the most common issues I discuss with my patients every day.

During this time your hormone levels are literally all over the show and blood tests are uninterpretable because they vary day to day so widely. Your oestrogen levels wobble like jelly, sometimes being too low but also sometimes too high, until two years before menopause when they really start to plummet. Unlike the yo-yoing oestrogen levels, progesterone levels also decline but do so gradually during perimenopause. Studies have shown that during perimenopause, the lower the progesterone level, the higher the likelihood of depression.

Brain fog of menopause. What is it?

Associate Professor Caroline Gurvich is Deputy Director of Monash Alfred Psychiatry Research Centre and head of the cognition and hormones group. 'I feel like it's [brain fog] a new term,' she told me, adding that when she trained as a neuropsychologist the term didn't exist at all. 'It's not a medical term.' Brain fog has also been reported with cancer chemotherapy and even after COVID-19.

What the experts do to maintain brain health
ASSOCIATE PROFESSOR CAROLINE GURVICH

Caroline exercises 30 to 60 minutes a day and that ticks a number of boxes for her, apart from fitness. 'My exercise is my self-care,' she says. It's also social time as she often exercises with a friend or as part of an exercise group. She adheres to a plant-based diet but for her that includes oily fish once or twice a week. She has one to two coffees a day and one to two glasses of wine with dinner a couple of times a week. Supplements are confined to vitamin D. 'That's only because a blood test showed I was deficient.'

As a full-time neuropsychologist, academic and mum of three, 'time is an issue'. So she has to prioritise. 'I'd like to find the time to meditate or do specific mindfulness practices,' she told me. But right now that's not practical. That doesn't mean her life has no pleasure. She puts a high value on connecting with friends and 'I always have a novel on the go'.

Given that brain fog is so common in perimenopause, we can kind of give you a fairly accurate descriptor based on the symptoms women report. 'It describes the fuzzy thinking that can come from lots of different places,' Caroline explained. 'In the context of menopause, it tends to include forgetfulness. Women forget why they came into a room, they say finding words is a problem and they forget names,' she added. Lots of women describe difficulty concentrating, 'not even being able to follow a TV or Netflix series,' she adds.

How common is it?

Figures vary. Julie Dumas is Research Associate Professor at the Clinical Neuroscience Research Unit of the University of Vermont, USA. 'Eighty per cent of women report brain fog,' she told me. That 80 per cent figure pretty much fits with my experience. When sitting with a new perimenopause patient, most are aware of, and often outright alarmed by, their brain fog.

What we know is that, as a rule, brain fog is a perimenopause problem and gets better as you cross the threshold into menopause proper. Let's say cheers to that! But that's not always the case.

What causes brain fog around perimenopause?

Professor Pauline Maki, whom we met in Chapter 8, has led much of the research into menopause and cognition, mood, and brain function in women. According to Professor Maki, studies consistently show that as a woman transitions from pre-menopausal to peri and then post-menopausal, her verbal memory declines sharply.

Are your hormones to blame or is it simply a matter of ageing? In a huge US study published in 2013, hormones were key. If you plotted memory against stage of menopause, the decline has a clear linear relationship with hormone levels that is clearer than the relationship between memory and age alone.

How long does brain fog last?

'We think it begins as soon as a woman's menstrual cycles begin to become irregular,' Professor Maki told the International Menopause

Society. 'Now when it goes away seems to depend. For some women it is absolutely time limited. When they transition through to post-menopause memory actually bounces back; we have very good data to suggest that. However, there do appear to be some women for whom the menopause transition represents a point in time at which their cognitive abilities decline a little bit and then kind of stay at that level.'

To explain this difference, Professor Maki says hormones clearly aren't the only reason. During the menopause transition you are getting falling oestrogen levels – albeit with a bit of zigzagging – on the way down. But after menopause, they pretty much plateau at negligible levels for every woman.

Caroline Gurvich says you need to look at brain fog in the context of what else is happening for a woman at this time of life. If she's having hot flushes, night sweats, insomnia and mood issues, they can make her brain feel very cloudy indeed. 'I think for anyone in the population, if you're not sleeping well, you're not thinking straight,' Caroline Gurvich pointed out.

Plus, as the various symptoms of peri and menopause take 10 years to get sorted, by the time they're over, your brain might be 10 years older so it can only rebound to the level it would have been at that age anyway, Caroline says.

Is it brain fog or incoming dementia?

Naturally lots of women who see me are experiencing brain fog and are terrified about what this means for their brains. Is this the beginnings of a dementing process?

Alzheimer's disease is exceptionally rare at the time most women go through menopause and peri, so it is unlikely to be anything more than menopause brain fog at this stage of life. As I have mentioned before, I like to say to my patients that if you lose your keys, you should consider it normal. But if you look at your keys and can't work out what to do with them, it's time to worry.

'The good news is that for the very, very, very, very large majority of women this has nothing to do with Alzheimer's disease,' Professor Maki said.

Having said that, see a doctor if you have brain fog plus you have or had a parent who had early onset dementia, which is defined as onset before age 60 (this could indicate a genetic link). Or if other people, such as close friends, colleagues and family members, are worried about your brain. If you feel that your brain fog is so bad that you can't work, again a proper assessment should be done.

What the experts do to maintain brain health
ASSOCIATE PROFESSOR JULIE DUMAS

Julie recommends exercising in groups with friends. She is part of a women's boot camp which she intersperses with running. 'It's social and it's aerobic,' she says. 'It's also my stress management.'

She takes a vitamin D supplement but this is due to the long Vermont winters spent mainly indoors. Other than that, she eats well, drinks alcohol a couple of days a week and doesn't avoid coffee.

How to battle brain fog

Here are my top tips for getting through the brain fog of peri and menopause.

- **Go easy on yourself**. At this time, more than ever, women can't expect cognitive perfection. We all make mistakes. Our brains cannot and should not be expected to be efficient all the time.

- **Don't just put up with hot flushes.** Here we are not talking about feeling a bit glowy once a day. But if your hot flushes make you uncomfortable and *especially* if they are taking out your sleep, get them sorted. That's because studies have found the worse your hot flushes, the worse you perform on memory tests. Ditto your sleep. See Chapter 9.
- **If you are experiencing depression, get it sorted.** Perimenopause is the highest risk time for women to experience a mood disorder. And depression not only interferes with your sleep, but your cognitive performance as well (see Chapter 8).
- **Control the things you can.** When things are a bit foggy upstairs, your great diet and exercise will be great friends! Control the things you can!
- **Remove distractions.** Most of us can only cope with so many distractions like ringing phones, email and text notifications, and Instagram pings. Silencing all those alarms and turning off notifications can really improve your focus.
- **Use compensatory cognitive strategies / External memory aids.** These can be super simple strategies to compensate for your brain being a little fuzzy. Caroline Gurvich says such strategies have been well studied for brain diseases from schizophrenia to traumatic brain injury. They're less studied for menopause brain fog but Caroline says many of her patients find them really helpful. Create a spot where you *always* leave your keys. Use your phone, Post-it notes, etc, for memory prompts. 'Use as much as you can to make your life as easy as possible,' she suggests.

Caroline pointed me to her colleague, Professor Elizabeth Twamley, Professor in Residence of Psychiatry at the University of California, San Diego. She specialises in neuropsychological assessment and cognitive rehabilitation and developed two linked programs called CogSMART (Cognitive Symptom Management and Rehabilitation Therapy) and CCT (Compensatory

Cognitive Training). 'They were originally developed for people with neuropsychiatric disorders who had mild to moderate cognitive impairments,' she told me. 'We know that neurological conditions, such as brain injuries and psychiatric illnesses, cause changes in the ability to attend, focus, learn and respond to information efficiently. Our goal was to help people implement cognitive strategies in their daily lives to more efficiently and effectively handle the cognitive demands they face.'

Some of the cognitive strategies taught through CogSMART and CCT help people handle cognitive demands in new ways. 'Some may be strategies that they already use, or have used in the past, but perhaps they need to make the strategy more automatic,' Professor Twamley said. When this happens, people end up implementing their preferred cognitive strategies so habitually that the strategies become part of the routine of daily life.

Many of the strategies are super simple. 'Making your daily activities into routines, making maximal use of your calendar system and a to-do list, talking out loud about what you are doing to improve task focus, and taking strategic breaks from demanding activities are a few of the strategies,' Professor Twamley suggested.

What the experts do to maintain brain health
PROFESSOR ELIZABETH TWAMLEY

Elizabeth uses all the CogSMART strategies herself. She says she is good at prioritising her sleep. 'As someone with two small children, I get a fair amount of physical activity,' she told me. 'But I would like to make more time for exercise, particularly to maintain muscle strength as I age.' She follows a plant-based diet, 'which is known to be associated with reduced cerebrovascular risk factors'.

Does HRT help brain fog?

The data is a bit all over the show at the moment because brain fog is a relatively recently described issue and it still isn't defined, making it hard to study. However, small trials say yes. At least for women in peri or younger post-menopausal women. In my practice, I am careful not to overpromise. For my patients, if HRT gets rid of hot flushes, helps a woman sleep better and helps her mood swings, her brain fog almost always improves. I'm not sure it's the effects of the hormones on her brain directly, but as long as we are all happy with the result, I don't really need to know . . . yet!

Does HRT help prevent dementia?

This is *really*, really complex. Professor Rebecca Thurston says that one of the issues is the length of time it takes between HRT being prescribed for menopause symptoms and the eventual development of cognitive impairment and dementia. 'You need long extended studies,' she points out. They're expensive. And by the time you get to the end of the study things might have changed. The women might now have high blood pressure, thyroid disease or diabetes.

Take the biggest ever study of HRT and health, the Women's Health Initiative. This is a massive long-term study funded by the National Heart, Lung and Blood Institute that began in the early 1990s and concluded in 2005, although extension studies are ongoing. It hit headlines all over the news in 2002 when one arm of the study that recruited women to either take HRT or a placebo reported that the HRT group had a higher risk of breast cancer. Women around the world chucked their HRT in the bin as horror headlines tried to outdo each other. When the study started, the average age of participants was 63 (who do you know that *starts* HRT at age 63?) and the type of HRT they took isn't really used any more. Not by any doctor who knows anything about menopause treatment. As an aside, the study data actually shows that there is no increased risk of breast cancer for women who start HRT when in perimenopause or just after menopause.

But the Women's Health Initiative also found that women aged 65 years and older who started HRT in the form of conjugated equine oestrogen and medroxyprogesterone for an average of four years *doubled* their risk of dementia. So, what I would take away from that is that regardless of what HRT can do for women who start taking it when in perimenopause, if you're already in your 60s or older, don't start HRT! That's certainly the recommendation of all menopause societies around the world.

What about when used correctly?

Studies show that women who start HRT early have better memory. MRI studies indicate that women on HRT have a bigger hippocampus. In 2021, a meta-analysis of 24 trials found that the majority of studies found that taking HRT reduced the risk of dementia by between 11 and 33 per cent, depending on the type of HRT taken and what it was taken for (e.g. symptom control).

Experts think that once you've been in menopause for a long time, the hormones in HRT won't help. But if HRT is started during that critical period right around menopause, they may well benefit the brain.

For now, we suggest that if you need HRT for control of hot flushes or other menopause symptoms, HRT might help your brain, too. But don't take it for brain protection alone as the evidence is just not there.

That is unless you went into early menopause (before age 45). If that's you, you should absolutely be on HRT until age 51 to protect your bones, heart and brain, too.

Testosterone and the brain

It's not just women who experience hormone-related brain changes. Testosterone affects the brain, too.

Testosterone, the main male hormone, is made by Leydig cells in the testes but also from adrenal hormones including dehydro-epiandrosterone (DHEA), androstenedione, androstenediol and androstenone. In the brain, it helps with the growth of new blood vessels, and powers up vascular remodelling, which maintains the health of blood vessels. It also prevents oxidative stress in the brain, helps maintain the integrity of the blood–brain barrier and generally protects the brain. In the hippocampus of the brain, testosterone can improve synaptic plasticity and prevent neuronal cell death. In rats, lower testosterone levels boost β-amyloid accumulation in brain neurons. Unlike women, who get a pretty dramatic drop in oestrogen levels around the time of menopause, testosterone levels in men drop more gradually. After the age of 40 years, men have a 1.6 per cent decline in testosterone levels each year.

Various studies have shown that men with low levels of testosterone perform poorly on tests of verbal fluency, visuospatial abilities, memory, executive function and attention. Studies in men with prostate cancer who have to take medications to suppress their testosterone levels to prevent cancer spread suggest that low testosterone levels might cause cognitive problems. And low testosterone levels have also been observed in patients with Alzheimer's disease and mild cognitive impairment.

Apart from a gradual decline with ageing, lots of super common chronic diseases can cause low testosterone levels. Conditions like type 2 diabetes, obesity, depression, obstructive sleep apnoea, chronic kidney disease or anorexia nervosa all cause low testosterone levels. In addition, certain medications, in particular steroids and opioid painkillers, are culprits.

Diagnosing low testosterone

I'm going to speak about Australia, where getting the diagnosis of testosterone deficiency is *sooooo* difficult, that lots of doctors give up. Men must complain of consistent symptoms and signs of testosterone deficiency (which are defined as reduced libido, decreased spontaneous erections, breast discomfort, loss of body hair, reduced shaving, very small or shrinking testes, infertility, height loss, low trauma fracture, low bone mineral density and hot flushes). *Plus*, there must be repeated low testosterone levels on early morning fasting blood testing.

Getting testosterone replacement therapy

In Australia, you need a men's health specialist or endocrinologist to confirm the diagnosis and start treatment. There are lots of ways it can be given. There are gels you rub on your forearm, a cream you can rub on your scrotum, injections and tablets. It's a matter of personal choice which one suits you best.

Researchers have tried using testosterone replacement therapy for men with low levels to prevent and treat cognitive impairment. Certainly there are trials that show that testosterone supplementation (50–100 mg of testosterone daily) boosts cognition and verbal memory and reduces symptoms of depression. But a 2019 meta-analysis of 23 trials found pretty depressingly negative results in relation to MCI and dementia. Many of the studies were small and conducted over a short period of time and on older men where the brain damage might already have begun.

The negative trials don't mean it's not worthwhile taking testosterone supplements if your levels are low and you have symptoms. It's just that we're lacking the evidence that it can help prevent dementia and MCI. So far. But before you head to your local supplier of choice, taking testosterone supplements is not without risks. These include increased risk of blood clots, prostate problems, breast enlargement, mood swings and aggression, decreased testicle size and worsening of sleep apnoea.

Takeaways

- At this stage you would *not* take HRT for prevention of dementia alone.
- But if you are taking HRT for hot flushes or other things, natural or micronised progesterone is better and transdermal oestrogen (patches and gels) are better than tablets.
- Same with testosterone replacement therapy for men.
- Meanwhile you can do lots of things to get your brain through this brain fog while your hormones are not playing nicely!

What the experts do

As I conducted the interviews for this book, I invited each expert to share what they do in their own lives to maintain their brain health and prevent cognitive decline. While each of them does something a bit different, there are also lots of similarities. Here is a summary of their feedback.

- Everyone exercises. And we're not talking slow strolling once a week. They do it properly.
- They all watch what they eat, but few are dogmatic about their diets, just generally going for a healthy diet with less junk food and processed foods.
- Nobody doesn't drink – except for reasons unrelated to brain health.
- They are all dedicated to getting 7–8 hours of quality sleep a night – well, as often as is practically possible.
- Only a couple of experts take brain supplements.
- All credit their work with keeping their brains cognitively active and with keeping them socially active.
- Most see a GP to get their vascular risk factors in check.
- None of them smoke.

These messages may be boring, but just *keep healthy*. It's not a secret magic pill, it's not an ancient mysterious cure – it's the stuff doctors say all the time, whether it's to help you prevent high blood pressure, diabetes, cancer or dementia. As Dr Trevor Chong so eloquently put it: 'People dismiss this advice as motherhood statements, like the GP just dishes this advice out because they have to say something, and they're sick of hearing it. But there's excellent evidence that this works.'

What the experts do

Thanks to all the medical professionals who contributed to this project.

Associate Professor Julie Dumas	Associate Professor, Clinical Neuroscience Research Unit, Department of Psychiatry, University of Vermont
Professor Ian Hickie	Co-Director of Health and Policy at the University of Sydney's Brain and Mind Centre
Associate Professor Hussein Yassine	Department of Medicine, Keck School of Medicine of the University of Southern California
Professor Ashley Bush	Head of the Oxidation Biology Unit and Director of the Melbourne Dementia Research Centre
Professor Rebecca Thurston	Pittsburgh Foundation Chair and Professor of Psychiatry, Psychology and Epidemiology, University of Pittsburgh
Dr David Perlmutter	MD board-certified neurologist, fellow of the American College of Nutrition, and five-time New York Times best-selling author of books including *Brain Wash*, *Grain Brain* and *Brain Maker*
Dr Michael Sughrue	Neurosurgeon and co-founder and chief medical officer at Omniscient Neurotechnology
Professor Rachel Buckley	Assistant Professor of Neurology at Harvard University and Massachusetts General Hospital
Professor Sharon Naismith	Chair of Psychology at the Charles Perkins Centre, the University of Sydney. She also heads the Healthy Brain Ageing Program at the Brain and Mind Centre.

Associate Professor Yen Ying Lim	Monash University Primary investigator of the Healthy Brain Project (healthybrainproject.org.au) and the BetterBrains Trial (betterbrains.org.au) Senior scientist at the Australian Imaging, Biomarkers and Lifestyle (AIBL) study
Associate Professor Caroline Gurvich	Deputy Director of Monash Alfred Psychiatry Research Centre and head of their Cognition and Hormones Group
Professor Victor Henderson	Professor of Neurology and Neurological Sciences at Stanford University and Director of the NIH Stanford Alzheimer's Disease Research Center
Dr Allen Orehek	Managing Director and founder of the Dementia Prevention Center in Pennsylvania Author of *Forget Alzheimer's: How to prevent Alzheimer's disease*
Dr Tim Sharp	Psychologist and founder of The Happiness Institute Author of *The Happiness Handbook*, and *100 Ways to Happiness: A guide for busy people*
Dr Loren Mowszowski	Clinical neuropsychologist and leader of the Cognitive Training research stream within the specialised Healthy Brain Ageing Program at the Brain and Mind Centre, the University of Sydney
Dr Trevor Chong	Cognitive neurologist and neuroscientist at the Turner Institute for Brain and Mental Health in Melbourne. He also leads the Monash Cognitive Neurology Laboratory.

What the experts do

Dr Joanna McMillan	Accredited practising dietitian, Adjunct Senior Research Fellow with La Trobe University, guest lecturer at the University of Sydney and a fellow of the Australasian Society of Lifestyle Medicine
Dr Raymond Schwartz	Neurologist and Clinical Associate Professor at the University of Sydney
Professor Elizabeth Twamley	Professor in Residence, Psychiatry, University of California, San Diego
Professor Dimity Pond	Professor of General Practice, Discipline of General Practice at the University of Newcastle
Professor Henrik Zetterberg	Professor of Neurochemistry at the University of Gothenburg, where he is the Head of the Department of Neurochemical Pathophysiology and Diagnostics. He is also the leader of the Fluid biomarkers for neuro-degenerative diseases group at University College, London.
Wayne Markman	CEO of Symbyx, a company that makes and sells infrared devices that claim to alter neuro-degenerative brain diseases by altering the gut microbiome through infrared light

To sum up

When I started writing this book, I was excited about the possibility of discovering the secret sauce for a young brain. Maybe there was a supplement I could take to undo the harm of sitting at my desk all day every day. Perhaps I could add some magic juice to my daily regimen, alongside my red wine and champagne, to split the difference?

But having interviewed 22 experts, dialled in to countless webinars and read close to 700 studies, I keep hearing the same things. There is *no* magic. There is no elixir of youth for the brain in the health food aisle of the supermarket or online. There are no expensive supplements or brain games that will work wonders. It comes down to basic good health with a big dose of common sense.

What is good for the heart is good for the brain. A healthy diet, a decent amount of exercise, drinking alcohol in the healthy range, keeping your blood sugar, blood pressure, weight, thyroid and cholesterol levels in the healthy range and getting enough sleep are key. Go to the dentist. Get your hearing checked and accept a hearing aid if you're going deaf. Look after your mental health; it is critical for your brain health. Use your brain, stay in the workforce if you can and be social. And have some compassion for your doctor. When they keep on repeating the message about healthy diet, and the need for regular exercise and sleep, it's not because they have run out of ideas about how to keep us healthy. It's because these things are the real deal!!

For me, the hardest change has been embracing exercise. I've had to make space for Tai Chi. It's a work-in-progress. I'm still going for bushwalks on the weekends. But I'm not beating myself up about it because so many of the other things on my 'healthy brain' list have tick marks against them.

Writing this book has been the most mentally challenging thing I have ever done. Thank you for coming on this journey with me. I wish you long and lasting brain health.

Acknowledgements

Thank you to my late nana. You were just the best grandmother. Thank you for leaving Poland, for fighting so hard for your family and for every warm hug and sloppy kiss, your Yiddish nursery rhymes and your chicken soup. I hope I told you enough when you were alive how much I loved you and still do.

Thank you to my late father-in-law, Louis. I wish I had known you before you started slipping away. But I thank you every day for creating the incredible human that is your son, Daniel. He is exactly the person that he describes you as! Smart, charming, quirky, considered, open-minded and curious. I know you loved and were proud of him, too.

Thank you to my late dad, Rodney. The thought of getting dementia horrified you. I lost you at 81 when your brain was 100 per cent intact. Dad, you never stepped off the pedestal you occupied my entire life. I miss your warmth, your wisdom and your wit every day. When the pain of your loss becomes unbearable, I tell myself how privileged I was to have had you as my father. There is no more grateful daughter in the world.

I also wanted to thank the brain experts who gave so generously of their time and expertise. Thanks to Professor Rachel Buckley, Professor Sharon Naismith, Dr Loren Mowszowski, Associate Professor Julie Dumas, Professor Ian Hickie, Professor Henrik Zetterberg, Dr Trevor Chong, Associate Professor Hussein Yassine, Professor Ashley Bush, Professor Rebecca Thurston, Professor Dimity Pond, Dr David Perlmutter, Dr Michael Sughrue, Associate Professor Yen Ying Lim, Associate Professor Caroline Gurvich, Professor Victor Henderson, Dr Allen Orehek, Dr Tim Sharp, Dr Joanna McMillan, Dr Raymond Schwartz, Professor Elizabeth Twamley and Wayne Markman.

Thanks also to the gun team at Murdoch Books, especially the incredible Sam Miles, who knew I was *dreading* the edit process and made it a dream! I also want to thank my manager, Simone Landes and as always, my incredible husband Daniel.

Endnotes

Introduction

1. *'And with over 55 million people living with dementia around the world as of 2022...'* Alzheimer's Disease International, https://www.alzint.org/about/dementia-facts-figures/dementia-statistics/

2. *'Modelling done by Dr Ron Brookmeyer, the Dean of the UCLA Fielding School of Public Health...'* Brookmeyer, R, Gray, S and Kawas, C. (1998). 'Projections of Alzheimer's Disease in the United States and the Public Health Impact of Delaying Disease Onset', *American Journal of Public Health*, Sept, Vol 88, No 9.

3. *'The fifth decade is the peak time for divorce in Australia.'* The Australian Bureau of Statistics. https://www.abs.gov.au/statistics/people/people-and-communities/marriages-and-divorces-australia/latest-release#divorces

Chapter 1

1. *'It accounts for 20 per cent of all of your body's oxygen consumption (more than any other organ)...'* Halliwell B. (2006) 'Oxidative stress and neurodegeneration: where are we now?' *Journal of Neurochemistry*, https://pubmed.ncbi.nlm.nih.gov/16805774/

2. *'... and sucks up 15 per cent of your heart's output...'* Tarantini S, Valcarcel-Ares MN, Toth P, Yabluchanskiy A, Tucsek Z, Kiss T, Hertelendy P, Kinter M, Ballabh P, Süle Z, Farkas E, Baur JA, Sinclair DA, Csiszar A, Ungvari Z. 'Nicotinamide mononucleotide (NMN) supplementation rescues cerebromicrovascular endothelial function and neurovascular coupling responses and improves cognitive function in aged mice.' *Redox Biology*, https://www.ncbi.nlm.nih.gov/pmc/articles/PMC6477631/

3. *'Glial cells are the rest of the brain's cells.'* Jäkel S and Dimou L (2017) 'Glial Cells and Their Function in the Adult Brain: A Journey through the History of Their Ablation'. *Frontiers in Cell Neuroscience*, https://www.frontiersin.org/articles/10.3389/fncel.2017.00024/full

4. *'Microglia are these amoeba-looking cells...'* Augusto-Oliveira M, Arrifano GP, Lopes-Araújo A, Santos-Sacramento L, Takeda PY, Anthony DC, Malva JO, Crespo-Lopez ME. (2019) 'What Do Microglia Really Do in Healthy Adult Brain?' *Cells*, https://www.ncbi.nlm.nih.gov/pmc/articles/PMC6829860/

5. *'But the attack mode can be excessive and actually cause damage to healthy brain tissue, not just the unwanted bugs or toxins.'* Stetka, B (2022) 'The cell that might trigger Alzheimer's disease', *Medscape Medical News*, https://www.medscape.com/viewarticle/967592?uac=117094MG&faf=1&sso=true&impID=4043900&src=WNL_infoc_220225_MSCPEDIT_microglia#vp_2

6. *'Astrocytes are essential for maintaining...'* Purves D, Augustine GJ, Fitzpatrick D, et al., editors. (2001) 'Neuroglial Cells' *Neuroscience. 2nd edition.* Sunderland (MA): Sinauer Associates, https://www.ncbi.nlm.nih.gov/books/NBK10869/

7. *'Oligodendrocytes are the cells that make...'* Bradl M, Lassmann H. (2010), 'Oligodendrocytes: biology and pathology', *Acta Neuropathologica*, https://link.springer.com/article/10.1007/s00401-009-0601-5

8. *'A healthy adult brain has about 100 billion...'* (2020), 2020 Alzheimer's disease facts and figures. *Alzheimer's and Dementia*, https://doi.org/10.1002/alz.12068

9. *'... neurons can live more than 100 years each.'* National Institute on Aging, (2017) https://www.nia.nih.gov/health/what-happens-brain-alzheimers-disease#:~:text=In%20Alzheimer's%20disease%2C%20as%20neurons,significant%20loss%20of%20brain%20volume.

10. *'Random fact: a male brain weighs about 1336 grams...'* Jawabri KH, Sharma S. [Updated 2022]. 'Physiology, Cerebral Cortex Functions'. In: StatPearls [Internet]. Treasure Island (FL): StatPearls Publishing, Available from: https://www.ncbi.nlm.nih.gov/books/NBK538496/

11. *'A whole stack of different studies have implicated the prefrontal cortex...'* Siddiqui SV, Chatterjee U, Kumar D, Siddiqui A, Goyal N. (2008) 'Neuropsychology of prefrontal cortex', *Indian Journal of Psychiatry*, https://www.ncbi.nlm.nih.gov/pmc/articles/PMC2738354/

Endnotes

12. *'Frontal lobe injuries classically cause . . .'* Siddiqui SV, Chatterjee U, Kumar D, Siddiqui A, Goyal N. (2008) 'Neuropsychology of prefrontal cortex', *Indian Journal of Psychiatry*, https://www.ncbi.nlm.nih.gov/pmc/articles/PMC2738354/

13. *'But studies based on functional MRI machines have found . . .'* Siddiqui SV, Chatterjee U, Kumar D, Siddiqui A, Goyal N. (2008) 'Neuropsychology of prefrontal cortex', *Indian Journal of Psychiatry*, https://www.ncbi.nlm.nih.gov/pmc/articles/PMC2738354/

14. *'The frontal lobes are critical to what we call prospective memory . . .'* Jawabri KH, Sharma S. [Updated 2022]. 'Physiology, Cerebral Cortex Functions'. In: StatPearls [Internet]. Treasure Island (FL): StatPearls Publishing, Available from: https://www.ncbi.nlm.nih.gov/books/NBK538496/

15. *'We know that in rats . . .'* Bass DI, Nizam ZG, Partain KN, Wang A, Manns JR. (2014) 'Amygdala-mediated enhancement of memory for specific events depends on the hippocampus', *Neurobiology of Learning and Memory*, https://www.ncbi.nlm.nih.gov/pmc/articles/PMC3888811/

16. *'. . . from a tiny study of people with epilepsy . . .'* Inman CS, Manns JR, Bijanki KR, Bass DI, Hamann S, Drane DL, Fasano RE, Kovach CK, Gross RE, Willie JT. (2018) 'Direct electrical stimulation of the amygdala enhances declarative memory in humans', *Proc Natl Acad Sci U S A*. https://pubmed.ncbi.nlm.nih.gov/29255054/

17. *'Studies have shown that if you stimulate the amygdala . . .'* Wright, Anthony (2020) 'Limbic system: Amygdala', https://nba.uth.tmc.edu/neuroscience/m/s4/chapter06.html

18. *'It is the earliest and most severely affected part of the brain . . .'* Anand KS, Dhikav V. (2012) 'Hippocampus in health and disease: An overview', *Annals of Indian Academy of Neurology*, https://www.annalsofian.org/article.asp?issn=0972-2327;year=2012;volume=15;issue=4;spage=239;epage=246;aulast=Anand

19. *'The tegmentum is a cluster of neurons . . .'* Kathleen Ruchalski, Gasser M. Hathout, (2012) 'A Medley of Midbrain Maladies: A Brief Review of Midbrain Anatomy and Syndromology for Radiologists', *Radiology Research and Practice*, https://doi.org/10.1155/2012/258524

20. *'Another mesh-like system running right through the brainstem is the spinothalamic tract . . .'* Iordanova R, Reddivari AKR. (updated 2021) *Neuroanatomy, Medulla Oblongata*. In: StatPearls [Internet]. Treasure Island (FL): StatPearls Publishing, Available from: https://www.ncbi.nlm.nih.gov/books/NBK551589/

21. *'. . . let me introduce the area postrema (aka the vomiting centre).'* Iordanova R, Reddivari AKR. [Updated 2021] *Neuroanatomy, Medulla Oblongata*. In: StatPearls [Internet]. Treasure Island (FL): StatPearls Publishing, Available from: https://www.ncbi.nlm.nih.gov/books/NBK551589/

22. *'There are some larger molecules, such as glucose, that can enter the brain through piggy backing onto specialised transporter proteins . . .'* Dash, Pramood, (2020) 'Blood Brain Barrier and Cerebral Metabolism', *Neuroscience Online*, https://nba.uth.tmc.edu/neuroscience/m/s4/chapter11.html#:~:text=Glucose%20from%20blood%20enters%20the,through%20the%20blood%20brain%20barrier.

23. *'The idea of the blood brain–barrier is to keep harmful toxins and bugs out but allow nutrients in.'* Gotz, J (2017) 'What is the blood-brain barrier and how can we overcome it?' *The Conversation*, https://theconversation.com/explainer-what-is-the-blood-brain-barrier-and-how-can-we-overcome-it-75454

24. *'I should point out that the brain has zero energy reserves . . .'* Hachinski V, Einhäupl K, Ganten D, Alladi S, Brayne C, Stephan BCM, Sweeney MD, Zlokovic B, Iturria-Medina Y, Iadecola C, Nishimura N, Schaffer CB, Whitehead SN, Black SE, Østergaard L, Wardlaw J, Greenberg S, Friberg L, Norrving B, Rowe B, Joanette Y, Hacke W, Kuller L, Dichgans M, Endres M, Khachaturian ZS. (2019), 'Preventing dementia by preventing stroke: The Berlin Manifesto.' *Alzheimer's and Dementia*, https://www.ncbi.nlm.nih.gov/pmc/articles/PMC7001744/

25. *'Cerebrospinal fluid (CSF) is the roughly 150 mls of fluid . . . around five times a day.'* Telano LN, Baker S. [Updated 2022 Jul 4]. 'Physiology, Cerebral Spinal Fluid'. In: StatPearls [Internet]. Treasure Island (FL): StatPearls Publishing, Available from: https://www.ncbi.nlm.nih.gov/books/NBK519007/

26. *'The glymphatic system also seems to help distribute . . .'* Jessen NA, Munk AS, Lundgaard I, Nedergaard M. (2015) 'The Glymphatic System: A Beginner's Guide', *Neurochemistry Research*, https://www.ncbi.nlm.nih.gov/pmc/articles/PMC4636982/

27. *'Neurotransmitters of the brain'* National Institute of Neurological Disorders and Stroke, (2022) https://www.ninds.nih.gov/health-information/patient-caregiver-education/brain-basics-know-your-brain#Image%201

28. *'Recently scientists have discovered that GABA helps with learning new information.'* Ruhr-Universitaet-Bochum (2015) 'Neurotransmitter GABA predicts learning.' *ScienceDaily*, www.sciencedaily.com/releases/2015/12/151210093032.htm

29. *'Serotonin is often called the "calming chemical" as it brings on sleep.'* Tully, K., Bolshakov, V.Y. (2010) 'Emotional enhancement of memory: how norepinephrine enables synaptic plasticity'. *Molecular Brain*, https://doi.org/10.1186/1756-6606-3-15

Chapter 2

1. *'But there has been a sea change in thinking.'* Sohn, E. (2018) 'How the evidence stacks up for preventing Alzheimer's disease', *Nature Outlook*, July, 559, S18–S20

2. *'Evidence is now mounting that 40–48 per cent of dementia risk is "modifiable"'.* Chong, Terence WH; Macpherson, Helen; Schaumberg, Mia, A; Brown, Belinda, M; Naismith, Sharon L, and Steiner, Genevieve Z. (2021) 'Dementia prevention: the time to act is now', *Medical Journal of Australia*, 214 (7).

3. *'Specifically, research in Australia shows that the modifiable risk factors include':* Chong, Terence WH; Macpherson, Helen; Schaumberg, Mia, A; Brown, Belinda, M; Naismith, Sharon L, and Steiner, Genevieve Z. (2021) 'Dementia prevention: the time to act is now', *Medical Journal of Australia*, 214 (7).

4. *'One study found that a 20-year-old is 75 per cent faster than a 75-year-old at substituting symbols for numbers.'* Queensland Brain Institute, The University of Queensland, Australia. https://qbi.uq.edu.au/brain/dementia/whats-difference-between-ageing-and   dementia#:~:text=As%20we%20age%2C%20our%20cognitive,but%20not%20exhibit%20obvious%20symptoms

5. *'Dementia is an umbrella term for symptoms caused by a loss of brain function . . .'* Greenblat, C. (2021) World Health Organization fact sheet, https://www.who.int/news-room/fact-sheets/detail/dementia

6. *'. . . if you look at any brain affected by Alzheimer's disease, you'll see a build-up of a toxic protein called β-amyloid . . .'* Alzheimer's Association (2020) '2020 Alzheimer's disease facts and figures', *Alzheimers & Dementia, The Journal of The Alzheimer's Association*, Vol 16, Issue 3. https://doi.org/10.1002/alz.12068

6a. *'Depression, paranoia, anxiety, apathy and irritability are also often early symptoms although . . .'* Gauthier S, Rosa-Neto P, Morais JA, and Webster C. 2021. World Alzheimer Report 2021: *Journey through the diagnosis of dementia*. London, England, Alzheimer's Disease International.

6b. *'There are often problems with language (such as trouble remembering common words) and visuospatial dysfunction . . .'* Quental NBM, Brucki SMD, Bueno OFA.(2009) 'Visuospatial function in early Alzheimer's disease: Preliminary study', *Dement Neuropsychol*, 3(3):234–240. https://www.ncbi.nlm.nih.gov/pmc/articles/PMC5618979/

7. *'Tau itself isn't always toxic. In fact, it is an important chemical in its own right . . .'* 'What happens to the Brain in Alzheimer's disease?' (2017) National Institute on Aging, https://www.nia.nih.gov/health/what-happens-brain-alzheimers-disease#:~:text=Neurofibrillary%20tangles%20are%20abnormal%20accumulations,to%20the%20axon%20and%20dendrites.

8. *'. . . who die with seemingly perfectly functioning brains but their autopsy reports . . .'* Isaacson, R; Culpepper, L; Zetterberg, H. 'Challenging Cases in Alzheimer's Disease: Applying Strategies to Inform Timely and Accurate Diagnosis', Medscape accessed July 2022. https://www.medscape.org/viewarticle/969018_2

9. *'The other ability that is affected early on in the disease . . .'* Chen, S.T; Sultzer, David, L; Hinkin, Charles, H; Mahler, Michael, E; Cummings, Jeffery, L. (1998) 'Executive functioning in Alzheimer's Disease', *The Journal of Neuropsychiatry and Clinical Neurosciences*, https://doi.org/10.1176/jnp.10.4.426

10. *'Every single cell in your body . . .'* Mulis, E; van Heel, D; Balkwill, F; Islam, K. 'Genes Made Easy', Genes & Health, https://www.genesandhealth.org/genes-your-health/genes-made-easy

Endnotes

11. *'And having a family history of . . .'* Loy, Clement T; Schofield, Peter R; Turner, Anne M; Kwok, John B; (2014), 'Genetics of dementia', *The Lancet*, 10.1016/S0140-6736(13)60630-3

12. *'Over 20,000 studies have been published on the genetics of AD so far . . .'* Ferdandez, F; Andrews, Jessica L. (2020) 'Genetics of dementia: a focus on Alzheimer's disease' *The Neuroscience of Dementia*, Vol 1, as accessed on ScienceDirect https://www.sciencedirect.com/science/article/pii/B9780128158548000094

13. *'But we know for sure about one rogue gene that definitely links to Alzheimer's . . .'* Hann, Mary, N; Mayeda, Elizabeth, R; (2010) 'Apolipoprotein E Genotype and Cardiovascular Diseases in the Elderly', *Curr Cardio Risk Rep* 4, 361–368. https://doi.org/10.1007/s12170-010-0118-4

14. *'It has no bearing on your dementia risk.'* (2019) 'Alzheimer's Disease Genetics Fact Sheet', National Institute on Aging, https://www.nia.nih.gov/health/alzheimers-disease-genetics-fact-sheet

15. *'. . . it turns out that this mutation might actually protect you . . .'* (2019) 'Alzheimer's Disease Genetics Fact Sheet', National Institute on Aging, https://www.nia.nih.gov/health/alzheimers-disease-genetics-fact-sheet

16. *'It also seems to bring the condition on earlier . . .'* (2019) 'Alzheimer's Disease Genetics Fact Sheet', National Institute on Aging, https://www.nia.nih.gov/health/alzheimers-disease-genetics-fact-sheet

17. *'. . . risk of developing Alzheimer's disease and dementia by between five and eight times.'* Queensland Brain Institute, University of Queensland, Australia. https://qbi.uq.edu.au/brain/dementia/genetic-risk-factors-dementia

18. *'. . . one study found the APOE e4 gene in 24 per cent . . .'* Slawsky ED, Hajat A, Rhew IC, Russette H, Semmens EO, Kaufman JD, Leary CS, Fitzpatrick AL. (2022) 'Neighborhood greenspace exposure as a protective factor in dementia risk among U.S. adults 75 years or older: a cohort study', *Environ Health*, 15;21(1):14. doi: 10.1186/s12940-022-00830-6. PMID: 35033073; PMCID: PMC8760791.

19. *'. . . but together these only account for between 5 and 10 per cent of early onset dementia.'* Jiao, B., Liu, H., Guo, L. *et al.* (2021) 'The role of genetics in neurodegenerative dementia: a large cohort study in South China', *npj Genomic Medicine*, https://www.nature.com/articles/s41525-021-00235-3

20. *'Scientists have found at least six mutations in the SNCA gene that seem to cause Lewy body dementia . . .'* (updated 2021 March), 'SNCA gene', *MedlinePlus*, https://medlineplus.gov/genetics/gene/snca/#synonyms

21. *'About 60 per cent of people with FTLD . . .'* Alzheimer's Association (2020) '2020 Alzheimer's disease facts and figures', *Alzheimer's and Dementia, The Journal of The Alzheimer's Association*, Vol 16, Issue 3. https://doi.org/10.1002/alz.12068

22. *'Overall, FTLD accounts for about 3 per cent of dementia cases . . .'* Hogan, D., Jetté, N., Fiest, K., Roberts, J., Pearson, D., Smith, E., . . . Maxwell, C. (2016). The Prevalence and Incidence of Frontotemporal Dementia: A Systematic Review. *Canadian Journal of Neurological Sciences / Journal Canadien Des Sciences Neurologiques, 43*(S1), S96-S109. doi:10.1017/cjn.2016.25

23. *'Up to 80 per cent of people with PD . . .'* UCSF Weill Institute for Neurosciences, Memory and Aging Centre, Parkinson's Disease Dementia, https://memory.ucsf.edu/dementia/parkinsons/parkinson-disease-dementia

24. *'. . . helping mRNA and DNA strands heal themselves . . .'* Mitra J, Hegde ML. (2019) 'A Commentary on TDP-43 and DNA Damage Response in Amyotrophic Lateral Sclerosis', *Journal of Experimental Neuroscience*, https://www.ncbi.nlm.nih.gov/pmc/journals/2511/#jen

25. *'Consequently, the cell's DNA is unable to repair itself.'* Mitra J, Hegde ML. (2019) 'A Commentary on TDP-43 and DNA Damage Response in Amyotrophic Lateral Sclerosis', *Journal of Experimental Neuroscience*, https://www.ncbi.nlm.nih.gov/pmc/journals/2511/#jen

26. *'This problem has been found in a stack of neurodegenerative diseases . . .'* de Boer EMJ, Orie VK, Williams T, *et al* (2021) 'TDP-43 proteinopathies: a new wave of neurodegenerative diseases' *Journal of Neurology, Neurosurgery & Psychiatry*, https://jnnp.bmj.com/content/92/1/86

27. *'In 2016, groundbreaking research using data from 1000 autopsies . . .'* James BD, Wilson RS, Boyle PA, Trojanowski JQ, Bennett DA, Schneider JA. (2016) 'TDP-43 stage, mixed pathologies, and

clinical Alzheimer's-type dementia'. *Brain*, https://www.ncbi.nlm.nih.gov/pmc/articles/PMC5091047/

28. *'At this point the condition only shows up on MRI scans when it is severe.'* Deng, F; Gaillard, F. (accessed on 21 Jul 2022) 'Limbic-predominant age-related TDP-43 encephalopathy (LATE)', Radiopaedia.org. https://doi.org/10.53347/rID-70377

29. *'The amyloid cascade hypothesis.'* Makin, Simon. (2018) 'The amyloid hypothesis on trial', *Nature*, 559, S4-S7 https://www.nature.com/articles/d41586-018-05719-4

30. *'Blood-brain barrier issues'.* Hachinski V, Einhäupl K, Ganten D, Alladi S, Brayne C, Stephan BCM, Sweeney MD, Zlokovic B, Iturria-Medina Y, Iadecola C, Nishimura N, Schaffer CB, Whitehead SN, Black SE, Østergaard L, Wardlaw J, Greenberg S, Friberg L, Norrving B, Rowe B, Joanette Y, Hacke W, Kuller L, Dichgans M, Endres M, Khachaturian ZS. (2019) 'Preventing dementia by preventing stroke: The Berlin Manifesto', *Alzheimer's and Dementia*, https://www.ncbi.nlm.nih.gov/pmc/articles/PMC7001744/

31. *'But, as the brain ages, the NMDA receptor system becomes progressively weaker.'* Newcomer JW, Farber NB, Olney JW. (2000) 'NMDA receptor function, memory, and brain aging' *Dialogues in Clinical Neuroscience.* 2(3):219-32. 10.31887/DCNS.2000.2.3/jnewcomer

31b. *'Inflammation on the brain'.* Jack CR Jr, Albert MS, Knopman DS, McKhann GM, Sperling RA, Carrillo MC, Thies B, Phelps CH. (2011) 'Introduction to the recommendations from the National Institute on Aging-Alzheimer's Association workgroups on diagnostic guidelines for Alzheimer's disease', *Alzheimer's and Dementia* Vol 7, https://doi.org/10.1016/j.jalz.2011.03.004

32. *'These include interleukin-1β, interleukin-6 (IL-6) and tumour necrosis . . .'* McGrattan AM, McGuinness B, McKinley MC, Kee F, Passmore P, Woodside JV, McEvoy CT. (2019). 'Diet and Inflammation in Cognitive Ageing and Alzheimer's Disease' *Current Nutrition Reports*, https://www.ncbi.nlm.nih.gov/pmc/articles/PMC6486891/

33. *'This sets up a cycle of inflammatory processes . . .'* Gu Y, Vorburger R, Scarmeas N, Luchsinger JA, Manly JJ, Schupf N, Mayeux R, Brickman AM. (2017) 'Circulating inflammatory biomarkers in relation to brain structural measurements in a non-demented elderly population' *Brain, Behavior and Immunity.* https://doi.org/10.1016/j.bbi.2017.04.022

34. *'Studies have found that people who experience brain fog after COVID . . .'* Zhou Y, Xu J, Hou Y, Leverenz JB, Kallianpur A, Mehra R, Liu Y, Yu H, Pieper AA, Jehi L, Cheng F. (2021) 'Network medicine links SARS-CoV-2/COVID-19 infection to brain microvascular injury and neuroinflammation in dementia-like cognitive impairment' *Alzheimer's Research and Therapy*, https://www.ncbi.nlm.nih.gov/pmc/articles/PMC8189279/

35. *'The idea here is that a combination of bad genes and bad lifestyle . . .'* Beishon Lucy; Panerai Ronney B., 2021 'The Neurovascular Unit in Dementia: An Opinion on Current Research and Future Directions', *Frontiers in Aging Neuroscience* vol. 13. www.frontiersin.org/articles/10.3389/fnagi.2021.721937

36. *'Early research points to the fact that people with a Factor V Leiden mutation . . .'* Bots ML, van Kooten F, Breteler MM, Slagboom PE, Hofman A, Haverkate F, Meijer P, Koudstaal PJ, Grobbee DE, Kluft C. (1998) 'Response to activated protein C in subjects with and without dementia: The Dutch Vascular Factors in Dementia Study', *Haemostasis*. https://www.karger.com/Article/Abstract/22432

37. *'This mutation, which is found in 1 in 20–25 Australians . . .'* Melbourne Haematology, http://www.melbournehaematology.com.au/fact-sheets/factor-v-five-leiden-mutation.html

38. *'Alzheimer's disease is thought to begin 20 years or more . . .'* (2020) 'Alzheimer's disease facts and figures', *Alzheimer's & Dementia*, Vol 16, issue 3, https://doi.org/10.1002/alz.12068

39. *'Symptoms of mild cognitive impairment include . . .'* Viggiano D, Wagner CA, Martino G, Nedergaard M, Zoccali C, Unwin R, Capasso G. (2020) 'Mechanisms of cognitive dysfunction in CKD'. *Nature Reviews Nephrology.* https://www.nature.com/articles/s41581-020-0266-9

40. *'According to different studies, anywhere between 3 per cent and 22 per cent . . .'* Zhao Y, Feng H, Wu X, Du Y, Yang X, Hu M, Ning H, Liao L, Chen H, Zhao Y. (2020) 'Effectiveness of Exergaming in Improving Cognitive and Physical Function in People with Mild Cognitive Impairment

Endnotes

or Dementia: Systematic Review'. *JMIR Serious Games*. https://www.ncbi.nlm.nih.gov/pmc/articles/PMC7367532/

41. '*... only 50 per cent of people diagnosed with MCI will go on to develop another type of dementia ...*' (2018) Rowe, Christopher, 'PET for Clinicians', Austin Health, University of Melbourne, https://www.ranzcp.org/RANZCP/media/Conference-presentations/SON%202018/Rowe_PET-for-Clinicians-Nov-2018.pdf

42. '*Here is the mega important bit: we know that the same risks for dementia are the same for ...*' Campbell NL, Unverzagt F, LaMantia MA, Khan BA, Boustani MA. (2013) 'Risk factors for the progression of mild cognitive impairment to dementia, *Clinics in Geriatric Medicine*. https://www.ncbi.nlm.nih.gov/pmc/articles/PMC5915285/

43. '*In one study set in general practices ...*' (1995) Callahan CM, Hendrie HC, Tierney WM. 'Documentation and evaluation of cognitive impairment in elderly primary care patients', *Annals of Internal Medicine*. https://pubmed.ncbi.nlm.nih.gov/7856990/

44. '*... researchers at the Mayo Clinic ...*' (updated 2021) Alzheimer's Association https://www.alz.org/media/Documents/alzheimers-dementia-tau-ts.pdf

45. '*However these drugs don't do much more than ...*' (2003) 'Memantine', *Australian Prescriber*, https://doi.org/10.18773/austprescr.2003.085

46. '*In 2022, SAGE-718, a new drug...*' 'Experimental drug may boost executive function in Alzheimer's' (2022) Burton, Kelli Whitlock, *Medscape Medical News*

47. '*In early studies the β-site ...*' (2019) Das B, Yan R. 'A Close Look at BACE1 Inhibitors for Alzheimer's Disease Treatment'. CNS Drugs. https://link.springer.com/article/10.1007/s40263-019-00613-7

48. '*In humans, six BACE1 inhibitors have now reached...*' (2022) Ricci, P. 'Medicinal chemistry in review: BACE1 inhibitors as a treatment for Alzheimer's disease', Domainex.co.uk, https://www.domainex.co.uk/news/medicinal-chemistry-review-bace1-inhibitors-treatment-alzheimers-disease

49. '*The results might have looked stellar on the scan ...*' Padda IS, Parmar M. (Updated 2022) 'Aducanumab', StatPearls Treasure Island (FL), StatPearls Publishing, https://www.ncbi.nlm.nih.gov/books/NBK573062/

Chapter 3

1. '*... scientists still have no good predictor ...*' Reiss AB, Glass AD, Wisniewski T, Wolozin B, Gomolin IH, Pinkhasov A, De Leon J, Stecker MM. (2020) 'Alzheimer's disease: many failed trials, so where do we go from here?' *Journal of Investigative Medicine*, https://jim.bmj.com/content/68/6/1135.long

2. '*In 2021, Alzheimer's Disease International released their World Alzheimer Report.*' Alzheimer's Disease International, McGill University (2021) https://www.alzint.org/resource/world-alzheimer-report-2021/

3. '*The updated UK dementia guidelines ...*' Alzheimer's Disease International, McGill University (2021), https://www.alzint.org/u/World-Alzheimer-Report-2021-Chapter-02.pdf

4. '*Dr Marshal Folstein first developed ...*' https://www.ihpa.gov.au/sites/default/files/publications/smmse-guidelines-v2.pdf

5. '*The General Practitioner Assessment of Cognition*'. http://gpcog.com.au

6. '*The Memory Impairment Screen.*' https://www.alz.org/media/Documents/memory-impairment-screening-mis.pdf

7. '*The Mini-Cog.*' https://mini-cog.com

8. '*The Addenbrooke Cognition Examination-Revised.*' César KG, Yassuda MS, Porto FHG, Brucki SMD, Nitrini R. (2017) 'Addenbrooke's cognitive examination-revised: normative and accuracy data for seniors with heterogeneous educational level in Brazil', *International Psychogeriatrics*, Vol 29, issue 8.

9. '*It takes about 20–25 minutes to do.*' *IPA Bulletin*, Volume 31, Number 3, https://www.ipa-online.org/news-and-issues/addenbrookes-cognitive-examination-revised-ace-r

10. '*The eight-item Informant Interview to Differentiate Aging and Dementia (AD8).*' https://www.alz.org/media/Documents/ad8-dementia-screening.pdf

11. *The Short Informant Questionnaire on Cognitive Decline in the Elderly (IQCODE)*' https://www.alz.org/media/documents/short-form-informant-questionnaire-decline.pdf

11a. *It has been* described as a moderately effective test with accuracy rates of between 60 and 74 per cent . . .' Ding, Y., Niu, J., Zhang, Y. *et al.* (2018) 'Informant questionnaire on cognitive decline in the elderly (IQCODE) for assessing the severity of dementia in patients with Alzheimer's disease.' *BMC Geriatrics*, Vol 18, article 146.

12. *The Montreal Cognitive Assessment (MoCA)*' *Dementia Care Central*. . .' (updated 2020) https://www.dementiacarecentral.com/montreal-cognitive-assessment-test/

13. *It is more accurate than the MMSE . . .*' Kang JM, Cho YS, Park S, Lee BH, Sohn BK, Choi CH, Choi JS, Jeong HY, Cho SJ, Lee JH, Lee JY. (2018) Montreal cognitive assessment reflects cognitive reserve. *BMC Geriatrics*, Vol 18, article 261

13a. *A 2015 review found that . . .*' Tsoi KK, Chan JY, Hirai HW, Wong SY, Kwok TC. (2015) 'Cognitive Tests to Detect Dementia: A Systematic Review and Meta-analysis', *JAMA Internal Medicine*, https://pubmed.ncbi.nlm.nih.gov/26052687/

14. *Routine blood tests help rule out conditions like diabetes . . .*' World Alzheimer's Report 2021, Alzheimer's International, https://www.alzint.org/u/World-Alzheimer-Report-2021-Chapter-08.pdf

15. *Scans are an awesome tool . . .*' Teng, L., Li, Y., Zhao, Y. *et al.* (2020) 'Predicting MCI progression with FDG-PET and cognitive scores: a longitudinal study' *BMC Neurology*, Vol 20, article148.

16. *Scans are not a predictor of future cognitive decline.*' Perdro, Rosa-Neto, *World Alzheimer's Report 2021*, Alzheimer's International, https://www.alzint.org/u/World-Alzheimer-Report-2021-Chapter-10.pdf

17. *. . . MRIs are better.*' Perdro, Rosa-Neto, *World Alzheimer's Report 2021*, Alzheimer's International, https://www.alzint.org/u/World-Alzheimer-Report-2021-Chapter-10.pdf

17a. *As a result, it is not the sort of scan . . .*' Wenwen Xu, Shanshan Chen, Chen Xue, Guanjie Hu, Wenying Ma, Wenzhang Qi, Xingjian Lin, Jiu Chen (2020), 'Functional MRI-Specific Alterations in Executive Control Network in Mild Cognitive Impairment: An ALE Meta-Analysis', *Frontiers in Aging Neuroscience*, https://pubmed.ncbi.nlm.nih.gov/33192472/

18 *That increased oxygen or sugar can be seen on the fMRI.*' Glover GH. (2011) 'Overview of functional magnetic resonance imaging', *Neurosurgery Clinics of North America*, Vol 22, Issue 2. https://doi.org/10.1016/j.nec.2010.11.001

19. *We're still working out . . .*' Wenwen Xu, Shanshan Chen, Chen Xue, Guanjie Hu, Wenying Ma, Wenzhan Qi, Xingjian Lin, Jiu Chen. (2020) 'Functional MRI-Specific Alterations in Executive Control Network in Mild Cognitive Impairment: An ALE Meta-Analysis' *Frontiers in Aging Neuroscience*, https://doi.org/10.3389/fnagi.2020.578863

20. *. . . you can actually see both β-amyloid and tau in the brain.*' Mary Beth Massat (2021) 'The Importance of Neuroimaging in Dementia Treatment' Applied Radiology, https://www.medscape.com/viewarticle/962140

21. *In studies, PET scans have been found to have a sensitivity of 80 per cent . . .*' Christopher Rowe, Austin Health, University of Melbourne, https://www.ranzcp.org/RANZCP/media/Conference-presentations/SON%202018/Rowe_PET-for-Clinicians-Nov-2018.pdf

22. *Measuring CSF β-amyloid 42 has . . .*' Blennow, K. (2017) 'A Review of Fluid Biomarkers for Alzheimer's Disease: Moving from CSF to Blood', *Neurology and Therapy*, Vol 6, 15–24.

23. *. . . the levels in CFS will st*art *to rise before . . .*' Alzheimer's Disease Neuroimaging Initiative, https://adni.loni.usc.edu/study-design/#background-container

24. *These CSF findings are already there in people . . .*' Blennow, K. (2017) 'A Review of Fluid Biomarkers for Alzheimer's Disease: Moving from CSF to Blood', *Neurology and Therapy*, Vol 6, 15–24.

25. *. . . CSF tau increases 20 years before dementia appears!*' Tahzeeb Fatima, Lennart T.H. Jacobsson, Silke Kern, Anna Zettergren, Kaj Blennow, Henrik Zetterberg, Lena Johansson, Mats Dehlin, Ingmar Skoog (2021), 'Association between serum urate and CFS markers of Alzheimer's disease pathology in a population-based sample of 70-year-olds' *Alzheimer's & Dementia*, https://doi.org/10.1002/dad2.12241

Endnotes

26. *'In fact, studies have shown that the false positive rate for diagnosis of mild cognitive impairment . . .'* Yu J, Xu W, Tan C, *et al, (2020),*'Evidence-based prevention of Alzheimer's disease: systematic review and meta-analysis of 243 observational prospective studies and 153 randomised controlled trials' *Journal of Neurology*, Neurosurgery & Psychiatry Vol 91:1201-1209.

27. *'Without any validated test, mild cognitive impairment is a clinical diagnosis . . .'* Ya-Xin Chen, Ning Liang, Xiao-Ling Li, Si-Hong Yang, Yang Ping Wang, nan-Nan Shi, (2021)'Diagnosis and Treatment for Mild Cognitive Impairment: A Systematic Review of Clinical Practice Guidelines and Consensus Statements', *Frontiers in Neurology*, https://doi.org/10.3389/fneur.2021.719849

28. *'And don't forget only 50 per cent of people. . .'* Christopher Rowe, Austin Health, University of Melbourne, https://www.ranzcp.org/RANZCP/media/Conference-presentations/SON%202018/Rowe_PET-for-Clinicians-Nov-2018.pdf

29. *'Having the APOE e4 allele increases your risk of dementia and seems to . . .'* Alzheimer's Disease Genetics Fact Sheet, National Institute on Aging, https://www.nia.nih.gov/health/alzheimers-disease-genetics-fact-sheet

30. *'People who have one copy of this APOE e4 mutation have a slightly higher dementia risk but people with two copies of APOE e4 . . .'* 'Genetic risk factors for dementia', Queensland Brain Institute, The University of Queensland, https://qbi.uq.edu.au/brain/dementia/genetic-risk-factors-dementia

31. *'After all, 24 per cent of people seem to carry . . .'* Slawsky, E.D., Hajat, A., Rhew, I.C. *et al.* (2022) 'Neighborhood greenspace exposure as a protective factor in dementia risk among U.S. adults 75 years or older: a cohort study', *Environmental Health*, Vol 21, https://doi.org/10.1186/s12940-022-00830-6

Chapter 4

1. *'Take the Finnish Geriatric Intervention . . .'* Kivipelto M, Solomon A, Ahtiluoto S, et al. (2013) 'The Finnish Geriatric Intervention Study to Prevent Cognitive Impairment and Disability (FINGER): study design and progress', Alzheimer's & Dementia, 9(6):657-65.

2. *'For the rest of the people in the study . . .'* 'A Multidomain Two-Year Randomized Controlled Trial to Prevent Cognitive Impairment- the FINGER study', Alzheimer's Prevention Organization, www.alzheimersprevention.org, https://wwfingers.com

3. *'After two years, the study has found that . . .'* https://wwfingers.com

4. *'In 2003, researchers conducted a meta-analysis . . .'* Colcombe S, Kramer AF. (2003) Fitness effects on the cognitive function of older adults: a meta-analytic study. *Psychological Science.*;14(2):125-30. https://doi.org/10.1111/1467-9280.t01-1-01430

5. *'Then in 2020, Taiwanese and US researchers . . .'* Chen, FT, Etnier JL, Chan KH, Chiu PK, Hung TM, Chang YK. (2020) 'Effects of Exercise Training Interventions on Executive Function in Older Adults: A Systematic Review and Meta-Analysis', *Sports Medicine*, 50(8):1451-1467. https://link.springer.com/article/10.1007/s40279-020-01292-x

6. *'In 2021, a US study of 180 people aged between 60 and 79 was published.'* Andrea Mendez Colmenares, Michelle W. Voss, Jason Fanning, Elizabeth A. Salerno, Neha P. Gothe, Michael L. Thomas, Edward McAuley, Arthur F. Kramer, Agnieszka Z. Burzynska,(2021) 'White matter plasticity in healthy older adults: The effects of aerobic exercise', *NeuroI Image*, Vol 239, https://doi.org/10.1016/j.neuroimage.2021.118305

7. *'But given that we know doing some kind of regular exercise . . .'* 'Benefits of physical activity' (2022) Division of Nutrition, Physical Activity, and Obesity, National Center for Chronic Disease Prevention and Health Promotion, https://www.cdc.gov/physicalactivity/basics/pa-health/index.htm Saint-Maurice PF, Coughlan D, Kelly SP, Keadle SK, Cook MB, Carlson SA, Fulton JE, Matthews CE. (2019) 'Association of Leisure-Time Physical Activity Across the Adult Life Course With All-Cause and Cause-Specific Mortality'. *JAMA Network Open*. 10.1001/jamanetworkopen.2019.0355 'Sleep Disorders' (updated 2021) Anxiety and Depression Association of America, https://adaa.org/understanding-anxiety/related-illnesses/sleep-disorders

7a. *'The case for exercise'* Johns Hopkins Medicine, https://www.hopkinsmedicine.org/health/wellness-and-prevention/7-heart-benefits-of-exercise

8. *'She pointed me to the results of the Dubbo Study of the Elderly . . .'* Simons LA, Simons J, McCallum J, Friedlander Y. (2006) Lifestyle factors and risk of dementia: Dubbo Study of the elderly. *Medical Journal of Australia.* https://pubmed.ncbi.nlm.nih.gov/16411871/

9. *'It also reduced the risk of ending up . . .'* McCallum J, Simons LA, Simons J, Friedlander Y. (2007) Delaying dementia and nursing home placement: the Dubbo study of elderly Australians over a 14-year follow-up. Annals of the New York Academy of Science. 10.1196/annals.1396.049

10. *'. . . this form of martial arts has benefits for muscle strength . . .'* 'Evidence-Based Program: Tai Chi for Arthritis and Falls Prevention', (2020), National Council on Aging, https://www.ncoa.org/article/evidence-based-program-tai-chi-for-arthritis-and-falls-prevention
    Zou L, Wang C, Chen K, Shu Y, Chen X, Luo L, Zhao X. (2017) 'The Effect of Taichi Practice on Attenuating Bone Mineral Density Loss: A Systematic Review and Meta-Analysis of Randomized Controlled Trials', *Int J Environ Res Public Health.* 10.3390/ijerph14091000
    Chao M, Wang C, Dong X, Ding M. The Effects of Tai Chi on Type 2 Diabetes Mellitus: A Meta-Analysis. J Diabetes Res. 2018 Jul 5;2018:7350567. 10.1155/2018/7350567
    Wang C, Schmid CH, Hibberd PL, Kalish R, Roubenoff R, Rones R, McAlindon T. (2009) 'Tai Chi is effective in treating knee osteoarthritis: a randomized controlled trial.' *Arthritis& Rheumatisim* https://onlinelibrary.wiley.com/doi/epdf/10.1002/art.24832

11. *'But a Chinese randomised prospective study . . .'* Mortimer JA, Ding D, Borenstein AR, DeCarli C, Guo Q, Wu Y, Zhao Q, Chu S. (2012) Changes in brain volume and cognition in a randomized trial of exercise and social interaction in a community-based sample of non-demented Chinese elders. Journal of Alzheimer's Disease, 10.3233/JAD-2012-120079

12. *'A 2021 study out of Singapore . . .'* Lee SY, Pang BWJ, Lau LK, *et al* (2021) Cross-sectional associations of housework with cognitive, physical and sensorimotor functions in younger and older community-dwelling adults: the Yishun Study *BMJ Open* 11:e052557. doi: 10.1136/bmjopen-2021-052557

13. *'This is called neuroplasticity, and is described in an article . . .'* Mateos-Aparicio Pedro, Rodríguez-Moreno Antonio (2019) 'The Impact of Studying Brain Plasticity' *Frontiers in Cellular Neuroscience,* Vol3. 10.3389/fncel.2019.00066

14. *'For example, studies show that doing cognitively stimulating . . .'* Stebbins RC, Yang YC, Reason M, Aiello AE, Belsky DW, Harris KM, Plassman BL. (2022) 'Occupational cognitive stimulation, socioeconomic status, and cognitive functioning in young adulthood' *SSM Population Health.* 10.1016/j.ssmph.2022.101024

15. *'Different studies have yielded wildly differing results and even meta-analyses of the various trials . . .'* Pergher, V., Shalchy, M.A., Pahor, A. et al. (2020) 'Divergent Research Methods Limit Understanding of Working Memory Training'. *Journal of Cognitive Enhancement,* Vol 4, https://doi.org/10.1007/s41465-019-00134-7

16. *'Some forms of cognitive training . . .'* Basak C, Qin S, O'Connell MA. (2020) 'Differential effects of cognitive training modules in healthy aging and mild cognitive impairment: A comprehensive meta-analysis of randomized controlled trials.' *Psychology and Aging.*

17. *'The ACTIVE trial has been going for over 10 years . . .'* Brain HQ, https://www.brainhq.com

18. *'But on objective testing . . .'* Rebok GW, Ball K, Guey LT, Jones RN, Kim HY, King JW, Marsiske M, Morris JN, Tennstedt SL, Unverzagt FW, Willis SL; (2014) 'ACTIVE Study Group. Ten-year effects of the advanced cognitive training for independent and vital elderly cognitive training trial on cognition and everyday functioning in older adults', *Journal of American Geriatric Society.* doi: 10.1111/jgs.12607.

19. *'For example, people who received reasoning and processing speed training . . .'* Souders Dustin J., Boot Walter R., Blocker Kenneth, Vitale Thomas, Roque Nelson A., Charness Neil.(2017) 'Evidence for Narrow Transfer after Short-Term Cognitive Training in Older Adults', *Frontiers in Aging Neuroscience,* Vol 9 https://www.frontiersin.org/articles/10.3389/fnagi.2017.00041

20. *'The ACTIVE trial has been criticised for being open to bias, as well as other issues . . .'* Kane RL, Butler M, Fink HA, et al. (2017) 'Interventions to Prevent Age-Related Cognitive Decline, Mild Cognitive Impairment, and Clinical Alzheimer's-Type Dementia' Agency for Healthcare Research and Quality (US).

Endnotes

21. *'In 2022, a Swedish meta-analysis . . .'* Gavelin HM, Dong C, Minkov R, Bahar-Fuchs A, Ellis KA, Lautenschlager NT, Mellow ML, Wade AT, Smith AE, Finke C, Krohn S, Lampit A. (2021) 'Combined physical and cognitive training for older adults with and without cognitive impairment: A systematic review and network meta-analysis of randomized controlled trials.' Ageing Res Rev. https://doi.org/10.1016/j.arr.2020.101232

22. *'In 2022, a Chinese meta-analysis looked at 10 studies . . .'* Zhao Y, Feng H, Wu X, Du Y, Yang X, Hu M, Ning H, Liao L, Chen H, Zhao Y. (2020) 'Effectiveness of Exergaming in Improving Cognitive and Physical Function in People With Mild Cognitive Impairment or Dementia: Systematic Review', JMIR Serious Games.

23. *'Research done at Johns Hopkins University . . .'* 'A league of your own', John Hopkins medicine, John Hopkins University, https://www.hopkinsmedicine.org/health/wellness-and-prevention/a-league-of-your-own

23a. *'There is consistent scientific evidence that living alone . . .'* Ingram J, Hand CJ, Maciejewski G. (2021) 'Social isolation during COVID-19 lockdown impairs cognitive function.' *Applied Cognitive Psychology* 10.1002/acp.3821

23b. *'. . . the evidence shows that socialising . . .'* Fratiglioni L, Wang HX, Ericsson K, Maytan M, Winblad B. (2000) 'Influence of social network on occurrence of dementia: a community-based longitudinal study', *The Lancet.* https://doi.org/10.1016/S0140-6736(00)02113-9

24. *'In February 2020, a new study from the Healthy Brain Project confirmed . . .'* Bransby L, Buckley RF, Rosenich E, Franks KH, Yassi N, Maruff P, Pase MP, Lim YY.(2022) The relationship between cognitive engagement and better memory in midlife. *Alzheimers Dementia* (Amst) https://doi.org/10.1002/dad2.12278

25. *'As you get older, owning a pet . . .'* Monica Shieu, Jennifer Applebaum, Galit Dunietz, Tiffany Braley (accessed July 2022), Companion Animals and Cognitive Health; A Population-Based Study', University of Michigan Medical Center, University of Florida.

Chapter 5

1. *'Despite this, a study published in 2022 . . .'* Long T, Zhang K, Chen Y, Wu C. (2022) 'Trends in Diet Quality Among Older US Adults From 2001 to 2018', *JAMA Netw Open*, 10.1001/jamanetworkopen.2022.1880

2. *'High fat and sugar diets can rapidly induce inflammatory changes . . .'* Beilharz JE, Maniam J, Morris MJ. (2015) 'Diet-Induced Cognitive Deficits: The Role of Fat and Sugar, Potential Mechanisms and Nutritional Interventions', *Nutrients*, https://www.mdpi.com/2072-6643/7/8/5307

3. *'A 2011 study showed that otherwise healthy university students . . .'* Francis HM, Stevenson RJ. (2011) 'Higher reported saturated fat and refined sugar intake is associated with reduced hippocampal-dependent memory and sensitivity to interoceptive signals', *Behavioral Neuroscience.* Dec;125(6):943-55. doi: 10.1037/a0025998. Epub 2011 Oct 24. PMID: 22023100.

4. *'A diet higher in saturated fats and refined sugar . . .'* Jacka, F.N., Cherbuin, N., Anstey, K.J. et al. Western diet is associated with a smaller hippocampus: a longitudinal investigation. BMC Med 13, 215 (2015). https://doi.org/10.1186/s12916-015-0461-x

5. *'Diets with a high DII score . . .'* Rajaram S, Jones J, Lee GJ. (2019) 'Plant-Based Dietary Patterns, Plant Foods, and Age-Related Cognitive Decline', *Advance Nutrition*, https://pubmed.ncbi.nlm.nih.gov/31728502/

5a. *'. . . rodent and human diets high in fat and refined sugar . . .'* Ramalho, A.F., Bombassaro, B., Dragano, N.R. et al, (2018) 'Dietary fats promote functional and structural changes in the median eminence blood/spinal fluid interface—the protective role for BDNF'. *Journal of Neuroinflammation* Vol 15, https://doi.org/10.1186/s12974-017-1046-8.

5b. *'Studies have confirmed that your gut microbiota . . .'* Maqsood R, Stone TW. (2016) 'The Gut-Brain Axis, BDNF, NMDA and CNS Disorders', *Neurochemistry Research.* https://pubmed.ncbi.nlm.nih.gov/27553784/

5c. *'Scientists are right now studying . . .'* Chong-Su Kim, PhD, Lina Cha, MS, Minju Sim, MS, Sungwoong Jung, MD, Woo Young Chun, PhD, Hyun Wook Baik, MD, PhD, Dong-Mi Shin, PhD

SAVE YOUR BRAIN

(2021) 'Probiotic Supplementation Improves Cognitive Function and Mood with Changes in Gut Microbiota in Community-Dwelling Older Adults: A Randomized, Double-Blind, Placebo-Controlled, Multicenter Trial', *The Journals of Gerontology: Series A*, Volume 76, Issue 1, https://doi.org/10.1093/gerona/glaa090

6. *'Studies have shown that in middle age . . .'* Beilharz JE, Maniam J, Morris MJ. (2015) Diet-Induced Cognitive Deficits: 'The Role of Fat and Sugar, Potential Mechanisms and Nutritional Interventions. *Nutrients.* doi: 10.3390/nu7085307. PMID: 26274972; PMCID: PMC4555146.

7. *'. . . and Dr Perlmutter pointed me to a study . . .'* Noh HS, Lee HP, Kim DW, Kang SS, Cho GJ, Rho JM, Choi WS. (2004) 'A cDNA microarray analysis of gene expression profiles in rat hippocampus following a ketogenic diet' *Brain Res Mol Brain Res.* doi: 10.1016/j.molbrainres.2004.06.020.

8. *'Ketones are available to the brain . . .'* Brandt J, Buchholz A, Henry-Barron B, Vizthum D, Avramopoulos D, Cervenka MC. (2019) 'Preliminary Report on the Feasibility and Efficacy of the Modified Atkins Diet for Treatment of Mild Cognitive Impairment and Early Alzheimer's Disease', *Journal of Alzheimer's Disease.* 2019;68(3):969-981. doi: 10.3233/JAD-180995. PMID: 30856112.

9. *'Back in the 1920s . . .'* Gano LB, Patel M, Rho JM. (2014) 'Ketogenic diets, mitochondria, and neurological diseases', *Journal of Lipid Research*, https://pubmed.ncbi.nlm.nih.gov/24847102/

10. *'There are now a few – albeit small – studies . . .'* Davis JJ, Fournakis N, Ellison J. (2020) 'Ketogenic Diet for the Treatment and Prevention of Dementia: A Review', *Journal of Geriatric Psychiatry and Neurology.* doi: 10.1177/0891988720901785.

10a. *'On a keto diet you would eat as few wholegrains . . .'* Vinciguerra F, Graziano M, Hagnäs M, Frittitta L, Tumminia A (2020). 'Influence of the Mediterranean and Ketogenic Diets on Cognitive Status and Decline: A Narrative Review, *Nutrients*, https://www.mdpi.com/2072-6643/12/4/1019

11. *'Increasing your sodium by 1–2 g a day may help.'* Anekwe CV, Chandrasekaran P, Stanford FC. (2020) 'Ketogenic Diet-induced Elevated Cholesterol, Elevated Liver Enzymes and Potential Non-alcoholic Fatty Liver Disease', *Cureus*, https://pubmed.ncbi.nlm.nih.gov/32064187/

12. *'The Mediterranean diet was first defined by Ancel Keys . . .'* Davis C, Bryan J, Hodgson J, Murphy K. (2015) 'Definition of the Mediterranean Diet; a Literature Review', *Nutrients*, Vol 7. https://www.mdpi.com/2072-6643/7/11/5459

13. *'This type of diet was found to be anti-inflammatory.'* Schwingshackl L, Hoffmann G. (2014), 'Mediterranean dietary pattern, inflammation and endothelial function: a systematic review and meta-analysis of intervention trials', *Nutrition, Metabolism & Cardiovascular Disease.* https://www.nmcd-journal.com/article/S0939-4753(14)00109-4/fulltext

14. *'A US study of 121 people . . .'* Aimee J Karstens, Lisa Tussing-Humphreys, Liang Zhan, Niranjini Rajendran, Jamie Cohen, Catherine Dion, Xiahong Joe Zhou, Melissa Lamar, (2019) 'Associations of the Mediterranean diet with cognitive and neuroimaging phenotypes of dementia in healthy older adults', *The American Journal of Clinical Nutrition*, Volume 109, Issue 2, https://doi.org/10.1093/ajcn/nqy275

15. *'One 2018 study of 116 older New Yorkers . . .'* Mosconi L, Walters M, Sterling J, Quinn C, McHugh P, Andrews RE, Matthews DC, Ganzer C, Osorio RS, Isaacson RS, De Leon MJ, Convit A. (2018) 'Lifestyle and vascular risk effects on MRI-based biomarkers of Alzheimer's disease: a cross-sectional study of middle-aged adults from the broader New York City area', *BMJ Open*, Vol 8, Issue 3.

16. *'And in 2013, a meta-analysis . . .'* Lourida, Ilianna; Soni, Maya; Thompson-Coon, Joanna; Purandare, Nitin; Lang, Iain A.; Ukoumunne, Obioha C.; Llewellyn, David J. (2013) 'Mediterranean Diet, Cognitive Function, and Dementia', *Epidemiology*, Vol 24, Issue 4.

17. *'. . . improves your chances of living a longer life in general . . .'* Guasch-Ferré M, Willett WC. (2021) 'The Mediterranean diet and health: a comprehensive overview', *Journal of Internal Medicine*, Vol 290, issue 3.

18. *'Studies show that the DASH diet . . .'* 'DASH diet to prevent and stop hypertension', The Royal Australian College of General Practitioners, Handbook of Non-Drug Interventions, https://www.racgp.org.au/clinical-resources/clinical-guidelines/handi/handi-interventions/nutrition/dash-dietary-approaches-to-stop-hypertension-diet

Endnotes

19. *'Studies also show that people who follow a DASH-type diet . . .'* Wengreen H, Munger RG, Cutler A, Quach A, Bowles A, Corcoran C, Tschanz JT, Norton MC, Welsh-Bohmer KA. (2013) 'Prospective study of Dietary Approaches to Stop Hypertension- and Mediterranean-style dietary patterns and age-related cognitive change: the Cache County Study on Memory, Health and Aging', *American Journal of Clinical Nutrition*, Vol 98, Issue 5.

20. *'Other studies show that switching . . .'* Tangney CC, Li H, Wang Y, Barnes L, Schneider JA, Bennett DA, Morris MC. (2014) 'Relation of DASH- and Mediterranean-like dietary patterns to cognitive decline in older persons', *Neurology*, Vol 14.

21. *'Like the DASH diet, the MIND diet isn't prescriptive . . . identifies five unhealthy food groups to avoid'*, Morris MC, Tangney CC, Wang Y, Sacks FM, Bennett DA, Aggarwal NT, (2015). 'MIND diet associated with reduced incidence of Alzheimer's disease', *Alzheimer's & Dementia*, Vol 11, Issue 9. https://www.ncbi.nlm.nih.gov/pmc/articles/PMC4532650/

22. *'Here is a comparison of the three diets that have ben studied. . .'* Morris MC, Tangney CC, Wang Y, Sacks FM, Bennett DA, Aggarwal NT, (2015). 'MIND diet associated with reduced incidence of Alzheimer's disease', *Alzheimer's & Dementia*, Vol 11, Issue 9. https://www.ncbi.nlm.nih.gov/pmc/articles/PMC4532650/

23. *'In one group of 6525 people . . .'* Anna Zhu, Hui Chen, Jie Shen, Xiaoxi Wang, Zhihui Li, Ai Zhao, Xiaoming Shi, Lijing Yan, Yi Zeng, Changzheng Yuan, John S. Ji, (2022), 'Interaction between plant-based dietary pattern and air pollution on cognitive function: a prospective cohort analysis of Chinese older adults', *The Lancet, Regional Health, Western Pacific*, Vol 20. https://doi.org/10.1016/j.lanwpc.2021.100372

23a. *'Placing mice and rats on a tight calorie-restricted . . .'* Pifferi, F., Terrien, J., Marchal, J. et al. (2019) 'Caloric restriction increases lifespan but affects brain integrity in grey mouse lemur primates', *Communications Biology* vol 1, https://doi.org/10.1038/s42003-018-0024-8

24. *'In humans . . .'* Kim CK, Sachdev PS, Braidy N. (2022) 'Recent Neurotherapeutic Strategies to Promote Healthy Brain Aging: Are we there yet?' *Aging and Disease*, Vol 13, issue 1. https://www.ncbi.nlm.nih.gov/pmc/articles/PMC8782556/

25. *'The research group released its latest findings in 2022'.* Kazumasa Yamagishi, Koutatsu Maruyama, Ai Ikeda, Masanori Nagao, Hiroyuki Noda, Mitsumasa Umesawa, Mina Hayama-Terada, Isao Muraki, Chika Okada, Mari Tanaka, Rie Kishida, Tomomi Kihara, Tetsuya Ohira, Hironori Imano, Eric J. Brunner, Tomoko Sankai, Takeo Okada, Takeshi Tanigawa, Akihiko Kitamura, Masahiko Kiyama & Hiroyasu Iso (2022) 'Dietary fiber intake and risk of incident disabling dementia: the Circulatory Risk in Communities Study', *Nutritional Neuroscience*, 10.1080/1028415X.2022.2027592

26. *'There is some evidence that people who are always a bit dehydrated . . .'* Watso JC, Farquhar WB. (2019) 'Hydration Status and Cardiovascular Function'. *Nutrients*, Vol 11. 10.3390/nu11081866

27. *'Women need to drink 2.1 litres . . .'* Australian Government National Health and Research Council, https://www.nrv.gov.au/nutrients/water

Chapter 6

1. *'Nicotinamide adenine dinucleotide (aka NAD$^+$) is a coenzyme essential for energy metabolism in the cell.'* Covarrubias, A.J., Perrone, R., Grozio, A.et al. (2021) 'NAD$^+$ metabolism and its roles in cellular processes during ageing.' *Nat Rev Mol Cell Biol* Vol 22, 119–141 https://doi.org/10.1038/s41580-020-00313-x

2. *'Studies show that lack of NAD$^+$ . . .'* Hong Weiqi, Mo Fei, Zhang Ziqi, Huang Mengyuan, Wei Xiawei, (2020). 'Nicotinamide Mononucleotide: A Promising Molecule for Therapy of Diverse Diseases by Targeting NAD+ Metabolism', *Frontiers in Cell and Developmental Biology*, Vol 8. https://www.frontiersin.org/articles/10.3389/fcell.2020.00246

3. *'NMN must be converted to NR to get into the cell . . .'* Hong Weiqi, Mo Fei, Zhang Ziqi, Huang Mengyuan, Wei Xiawei, (2020). 'Nicotinamide Mononucleotide: A Promising Molecule for Therapy of Diverse Diseases by Targeting NAD+ Metabolism', *Frontiers in Cell and Developmental Biology*, Vol 8. https://www.frontiersin.org/articles/10.3389/fcell.2020.00246

4. *'There are a ton of studies . . .'* Harshani Nadeeshani, Jinyao Li, Tianlei Ying, Baohong Zhang, Jun Lu. (2022) 'Nicotinamide mononucleotide (NMN) as an anti-aging health product – Promises and safety concerns', *Journal of Advanced Research*, Vol 37, 267-278, https://www.sciencedirect.com/science/article/pii/S2090123221001491

5. *'It is thought to help with athletic performance . . .'* Benameur T, Soleti R, Porro C. (2021) 'The Potential Neuroprotective Role of Free and Encapsulated Quercetin Mediated by miRNA against Neurological Diseases', *Nutrients*, Vol 16. https://www.ncbi.nlm.nih.gov/pmc/articles/PMC8073422/

6. *'In addition to this . . .'* Holland TM, Agarwal P, Wang Y, Leurgans SE, Bennett DA, Booth SL, Morris MC. (2020) 'Dietary flavonols and risk of Alzheimer dementia', *Neurology*, Vol 94. https://www.ncbi.nlm.nih.gov/pmc/articles/PMC7282875/

7. *'Studies using cell cultures . . .'* Breuss JM, Atanasov AG, Uhrin P. (2019) 'Resveratrol and Its Effects on the Vascular System', *International Journal of Molecular Sciences*, Vol 27. https://www.ncbi.nlm.nih.gov/pmc/articles/PMC6479680/

8. *'Sirtuins are proteins . . .'* Kane AE, and Sinclair DA, (2018) 'Sirtuins and NAD$^+$ in the Development and Treatment of Metabolic and Cardiovascular Diseases', *Circulation Research*, Vol 123. https://www.ahajournals.org/doi/full/10.1161/CIRCRESAHA.118.312498

9. *'. . . improved the health of several species of mice.'* Grabowska W, Sikora E, Bielak-Zmijewska A. (2017) 'Sirtuins, a promising target in slowing down the ageing process'. *Biogerontology*, Vol 18. https://www.ncbi.nlm.nih.gov/pmc/articles/PMC5514220/

10. *'There are human studies . . .'* Gomes BAQ, Silva JPB, Romeiro CFR, Dos Santos SM, Rodrigues CA, Gonçalves PR, Sakai JT, Mendes PFS, Varela ELP, Monteiro MC. (2018) 'Neuroprotective Mechanisms of Resveratrol in Alzheimer's Disease: Role of SIRT1'. *Oxidative Medicine and Cellular Longevity*, Vol 2018. https://www.hindawi.com/journals/omcl/2018/8152373/

11. *'A six-month study . . .'* Witte AV, Kerti L, Margulies DS, Flöel A. (2014) Effects of resveratrol on memory performance, hippocampal functional connectivity, and glucose metabolism in healthy older adults. *Journal of Neuroscience*. https://www.ncbi.nlm.nih.gov/pmc/articles/PMC6608268/

12. *'On the other hand, a study in 60 young adults . . .'* Wightman EL, Haskell-Ramsay CF, Reay JL, Williamson G, Dew T, Zhang W, Kennedy DO. (2015) 'The effects of chronic trans-resveratrol supplementation on aspects of cognitive function, mood, sleep, health and cerebral blood flow in healthy, young humans', *British Journal Nutrition*, Vol 114.

13. *'. . . a placebo-controlled trial . . .'* Thaung Zaw JJ, Howe PRC, Wong RHX (2020). 'Sustained Cerebrovascular and Cognitive Benefits of Resveratrol in Postmenopausal Women', *Nutrients*, https://www.mdpi.com/2072-6643/12/3/828

14. *'Two studies of the effects of anaesthetics . . .'* Popescu A, German M. Vitamin K2 Holds Promise for Alzheimer's Prevention and Treatment', (2021). *Nutrients*. https://www.mdpi.com/2072-6643/13/7/2206

15. *'. . . low consumption of vitamin K1 in the diet . . .'* Carrié I, Bélanger E, Portoukalian J, Rochford J, Ferland G. (2011) 'Lifelong low-phylloquinone intake is associated with cognitive impairments in old rats', *Journal of Nutrition*, Issue 8. https://academic.oup.com/jn/article/141/8/1495/4630529

16. *'One Irish study . . .'* Kiely A, Ferland G, Ouliass B, O'Toole PW, Purtill H, O'Connor EM. (2023) Vitamin K status and inflammation are associated with cognition in older Irish adults. *Nutritional Neuroscience*, Vol 23. https://www.tandfonline.com/doi/full/10.1080/10284 15X.2018.1536411

17. *'. . . in a study of 599 participants . . .'* van den Heuvel EG, van Schoor NM, Vermeer C, Zwijsen RM, den Heijer M, Comijs HC. (2015) 'Vitamin K Status Is not Associated with Cognitive Decline in Middle Aged Adults' *Journal of Nutrition, Health and Aging*, Vol 19. https://link.springer.com/article/10.1007/s12603-015-0579-8

18. *'For a start, some (but certainly not all) . . .'* 'Omega-3 Fatty Acids' National Institutes of Health, Dietary SupplementFactSheet, https://ods.od.nih.gov/factsheets/Omega3FattyAcids-HealthProfessional/

Endnotes

19. *'Your body uses omega-3s to make key signalling . . .'* Tassoni D, Kaur G, Weisinger RS, Sinclair AJ. (2008) The role of eicosanoids in the brain. Asia Pacific Journal of Clinical Nutrition. Vol 17. PMID: 18296342

20. *'Results from clinical trials . . .'* Drover, J., Hoffman, D.R., Castañeda, Y.S., Morale, S.E. and Birch, E.E. (2009), 'Three Randomized Controlled Trials of Early Long-Chain Polyunsaturated Fatty Acid Supplementation on Means-End Problem Solving in 9-Month-Olds', *Child Development*, 80: 1376-1384. https://doi.org/10.1111/j.1467-8624.2009.01339.x

21. *'Curcumin, the active ingredient in turmeric . . .'* Sandur SK, Pandey MK, Sung B, Ahn KS, Murakami A, Sethi G, Limtrakul P, Badmaev V, Aggarwal BB. (2007) 'Curcumin, demethoxycurcumin, bisdemethoxycurcumin, tetrahydrocurcumin and turmerones differentially regulate anti-inflammatory and anti-proliferative responses through a ROS-independent mechanism', *Carcinogenesis*. https://pubmed.ncbi.nlm.nih.gov/17522064/

22. *'It also has been shown to have anti-inflammatory and neuroprotective . . .'* Aggarwal BB, Harikumar KB. (2009) Potential therapeutic effects of curcumin, the anti-inflammatory agent, against neurodegenerative, cardiovascular, pulmonary, metabolic, autoimmune and neoplastic diseases. *International Journal of Biochemistry and Cell Biology*. https://link.springer.com/chapter/10.1007/978-0-387-46401-5_8

23. *'Studies in rats . . .'* Sarker MR, Franks SF. (2018) 'Efficacy of curcumin for age-associated cognitive decline: a narrative review of preclinical and clinical studies', *Geroscience*. Vol 40. https://link.springer.com/article/10.1007/s11357-018-0017

24. *'High homocysteine levels have been . . .'* Malouf R, Grimley Evans J, Areosa Sastre A. (2003) 'Folic acid with or without vitamin B12 for cognition and dementia' *Cochrane Database of Systematic Reviews*, Issue 4. Accessed 02 August 2022. https://www.cochranelibrary.com/cdsr/doi/10.1002/14651858.CD004514/full

25. *'However, when this was studied by a 2008 Cochrane review . . .'* Malouf R, Grimley Evans J. (2008) 'Folic acid with or without vitamin B12 for the prevention and treatment of healthy elderly and demented people', *Cochrane Database of Systematic Reviews* Issue 4. Accessed 02 August 2022. https://www.cochranelibrary.com/cdsr/doi/10.1002/14651858.CD004514.pub2/full

26. *'Vitamin B12, Vitamin B6 and folic acid help break down homocysteine . . .'* https://medlineplus.gov/lab-tests/homocysteine-test/

27. *'In 2018, a Cochrane review . . .'* Rutjes AW, Denton DA, Di Nisio M, Chong LY, Abraham RP, Al-Assaf AS, Anderson JL, Malik MA, Vernooij RW, Martínez G, Tabet N, McCleery J. 'Vitamin and mineral supplementation for maintaining cognitive function in cognitively healthy people in mid and late life', Cochrane Database System Review. doi: https://www.cochranelibrary.com/cdsr/doi/10.1002/14651858.CD011906.pub2/full

28. *'The massive COSMOS trial (COcoa Supplement and Multivitamin Outcomes Study) . . .'* https://cosmostrial.org/results/

29. *'A spin-off study . . .'* https://clinicaltrials.gov/ct2/show/record/NCT03035201

30. *'It was found that the older participants . . .'* https://www.whi.org/md/news/cosmos-mind-results

31. *'. . . and both the production and breakdown of neurotransmitters . . .'* Hosking DE, Ayton S, Beckett N, Booth A, Peters R. (2018) 'More evidence is needed. Iron, incident cognitive decline and dementia: a systematic review', *Therapeutic Advances in Chronic Disease*, https://www.ncbi.nlm.nih.gov/pmc/articles/PMC6348531/

32. *'. . . lower zinc levels . . .'* Squitti R, Pal A, Picozza M, Avan A, Ventriglia M, Rongioletti MC, Hoogenraad T. (2020) 'Zinc Therapy in Early Alzheimer's Disease: Safety and Potential Therapeutic Efficacy', *Biomolecules*. https://www.ncbi.nlm.nih.gov/pmc/articles/PMC7466035/

33. *'Studies have shown that people with Alzheimer's disease . . .'* Ventriglia M, Brewer GJ, Simonelli I, Mariani S, Siotto M, Bucossi S, Squitti R. (2015) 'Zinc in Alzheimer's Disease: A Meta-Analysis of Serum, Plasma, and Cerebrospinal Fluid Studies', *Journal of Alzheimer's Disease*, 2015;46(1): 75-87. doi: 10.3233/JAD-141924. PMID: 25697706.

34. *'Worse, in mice, excessive zinc supplementation . . .'* Liu F, Zhang Z, Zhang L, Meng RN, Gao J, Jin M, Li M, Wang XP. (2022) 'Effect of metal ions on Alzheimer's disease', *Brain Behaviour*.

Mar;12(3):e2527. doi: 10.1002/brb3.2527. Epub 2022 Feb 24. PMID: 35212185; PMCID: PMC8933773.

35. *'A Brazilian study identified that, in men at least . . .'* Benseñor, I.M., Lotufo, P.A., Menezes, P.R. et al. (2010) 'Subclinical hyperthyroidism and dementia: the Sao Paulo Ageing & Health Study' (SPAH). *BMC Public Health* Vol 10, 298. https://doi.org/10.1186/1471-2458-10-298

36. *'Iodine deficiency is the biggest cause of thyroid problems . . .'* The Australian Thyroid Foundation, https://www.thyroidfoundation.org.au/Iodine-Deficiency#:~:text=What%20is%20 Iodine%20Deficiency%3F,and%20neurodevelopmental%20disorders%20in%20newborns.

37. *'The rationale for taking vitamin E supplements to prevent and treat dementia . . .'* Browne D, McGuinness B, Woodside JV, McKay GJ. (2019) 'Vitamin E and Alzheimer's disease: what do we know so far?' *Clinical Interventions in Aging*, Jul, Vol 18, https://doi.org/10.2147/CIA.S186760

38. *'It looks like diets high in vitamin E do help prevent dementia.'* Browne D, McGuinness B, Woodside JV, McKay GJ. (2019) 'Vitamin E and Alzheimer's disease: what do we know so far?' *Clinical Interventions in Aging*, Jul, Vol 18, https://doi.org/10.2147/CIA.S186760

39. *'A 2017 Cochrane review found no evidence that the vitamin helps prevent people developing dementia . . .'* Farina N, Llewellyn D, Isaac MGEKN, Tabet N. (2017) 'Vitamin E for Alzheimer's dementia and mild cognitive impairment'. Cochrane Database of Systematic Reviews 2017, Issue 4. Art. https://doi.org/10.1002/14651858.CD002854.pub5. Accessed 18 August 2022.

40. *'Plus studies show that vitamin E supplements might increase the risk of a haemorrhagic . . .'* Schürks M, Glynn RJ, Rist PM, Tzourio C, Kurth T. (2010) 'Effects of vitamin E on stroke subtypes: meta-analysis of randomised controlled trials', *BMJ*, Nov, https://doi.org/10.1136/bmj.c5702

41. *'A study published in 2022 . . .'* May A. Beydoun, Hind A. Beydoun, Marie T. Fanelli-Kuczmarski, Jordan Weiss, Sharmin Hossain, Jose Atilio Canas, Michele KimEvans, Alan B. Zonderman (2022) 'Association of Serum Antioxidant Vitamins and Carotenoids With Incident Alzheimer Disease and All-Cause Dementia Among US Adults' *Neurology*, May, Vol 98. https://doi.org/10.1212/WNL.0000000000200289

42. *'The Ginkgo Evaluation of Memory (GEM) study . . .'* The National Center for Complementary and Integrative Health, https://www.nccih.nih.gov/health/the-ginkgo-evaluation-of-memory-gem-study

43. *'That said, a company-sponsored review of EGb 761 . . .'* Kandiah N, Chan YF, Chen C, Dasig D, Dominguez J, Han SH, Jia J, Kim S, Limpawattana P, Ng LL, Nguyen DT, Ong PA, Raya-Ampil E, Saedon N, Senanarong V, Setiati S, Singh H, Suthisisang C, Trang TM, Turana Y, Venketasubramanian N, Yong FM, Youn YC, Ihl R. (2021) 'Strategies for the use of Ginkgo biloba extract, EGb 761®, in the treatment and management of mild cognitive impairment in Asia: Expert consensus.' *CNS Neuroscience and Therapeutics*, Vol 27. https://www.ncbi.nlm.nih. gov/pmc/articles/PMC7816207/

44. *'People with Alzheimer's have less of the bugs known as Firmicutes and Bifidobacterium, but an increase in other bugs called Bacteroidetes.'* Vogt, N.M., Kerby, R.L., Dill-McFarland, K.A. et al. (2017) 'Gut microbiome alterations in Alzheimer's disease', Scientific Reports Vol 7, https://doi.org/10.1038/s41598-017-13601-y

45. *'This imbalance impacts on some of the inflammatory pathways in the gut and is measurable in the blood-stream.'* Sharma, Vivek Kumar, Thakur Gurjeet Singh, Nikhil Garg, Sonia Dhiman, Saurabh Gupta, Md. Habibur Rahman, Agnieszka Najda, Magdalena Walasek-Janusz, Mohamed Kamel, Ghadeer M. Albadrani, Muhammad Furqan Akhtar, Ammara Saleem, Ahmed E. Altyar, and Mohamed M. Abdel-Daim. 2021. 'Dysbiosis and Alzheimer's Disease: A Role for Chronic Stress?' *Biomolecules* 11, no. 5: 678. https://doi.org/10.3390/biom11050678

46. *'He pointed to some studies in rodents with dementia . . .'* Imran Khan, Sabrina Pathan, Xiao Ang Li, Wai Kit Leong, Wei Lin Liao, Vincent Wong, W.L. Wendy Hsiao, (2020), 'Far infrared radiation induces changes in gut microbiota and activates GPCRs in mice', *Journal of Advanced Research*, Volume 22, Pages 145-152, https://doi.org/10.1016/j.jare.2019.12.003

47. *'A 2020 Cochrane review of treatment with Souvenaid looked at three randomised . . .'* Burckhardt M, Watzke S, Wienke A, Langer G, Fink A. (2020) 'Souvenaid for Alzheimer's disease' Cochrane Database System Review. https://www.ncbi.nlm.nih.gov/pmc/articles/PMC8094446/

Endnotes

48. '*In 2019, a large US trial was published in the* Journal of the American Medical Association . . .' Koch M, Fitzpatrick AL, Rapp SR, Nahin RL, Williamson JD, Lopez OL, DeKosky ST, Kuller LH, Mackey RH, Mukamal KJ, Jensen MK, Sink KM. (2019) 'Alcohol Consumption and Risk of Dementia and Cognitive Decline Among Older Adults With or Without Mild Cognitive Impairment', *Journal of the American Medical Association*, https://www.ncbi.nlm.nih.gov/pmc/articles/PMC6777245/

49. '*Heavy alcohol abuse . . .*' Dementia Australia, https://www.dementia.org.au/about-dementia/types-of-dementia/alcohol-related-dementia

50. '*Well, similar benefits were found in a cohort of Norwegians, who were aged 60 plus.*' Johnsen B, Strand BH, Martinaityte I, Mathiesen EB, Schirmer H. (2021), 'Improved Cognitive Function in the Tromsø Study in Norway From 2001 to 2016', *Neurology Clinical Practise*. https://pubmed.ncbi.nlm.nih.gov/34992969/

51. '*But my favourite study is the home-grown Dubbo Study of the Elderly.*' Simons LA, Simons J, McCallum J, Friedlander Y. (2006) 'Lifestyle factors and risk of dementia: Dubbo Study of the elderly', *Medical Journal of Australia*.

52. '*In 2018, a meta-analysis of eight different studies was published.*' Larsson SC, Orsini N. (2018) 'Coffee Consumption and Risk of Dementia and Alzheimer's Disease: A Dose-Response Meta-Analysis of Prospective Studies', *Nutrients*, https://www.mdpi.com/2072-6643/10/10/1501

53. 'But *in 2021, data from the enormous UK Biobank was more conclusive.*' Zhang Y, Yang H, Li S, Li WD, Wang Y. (2121) 'Consumption of coffee and tea and risk of developing stroke, dementia, and poststroke dementia: A cohort study in the UK Biobank', *PLOS Medicine*, https://journals.plos.org/plosmedicine/article?id=10.1371/journal.pmed.1003830

Chapter 7

1. '*That's because US data shows that almost half of all US adults aged 45 and older . . .*' Omura JD, McGuire LC, Patel R, et al. (2022), 'Modifiable Risk Factors for Alzheimer Disease and Related Dementias Among Adults Aged ≥45 Years — United States', Morbidity and Mortality Weekly Report http://dx.doi.org/10.15585/mmwr.mm7120a2

2. '*A massive meta-analysis of studies was done in 2017 . . .*' Livingston G, Huntley J, Sommerlad A, Ames D, Ballard C, Banerjee S, Brayne C, Burns A, Cohen-Mansfield J, Cooper C, Costafreda SG, Dias A, Fox N, Gitlin LN, Howard R, Kales HC, Kivimäki M, Larson EB, Ogunniyi A, Orgeta V, Ritchie K, Rockwood K, Sampson EL, Samus Q, Schneider LS, Selbæk G, Teri L, Mukadam N. (2020) 'Dementia prevention, intervention, and care: 2020 report of the Lancet Commission'. *Lancet*, Aug 8;396 (10248):413-446. https://www.thelancet.com/journals/lancet/article/PIIS0140-6736(20)30367-6/fulltext

3. '*A 25-year prospective study of 3777 people aged 65 years or older . . .*' Amieva H, Ouvrard C, Meillon C, Rullier L, Dartigues JF, (2018) 'Death, Depression, Disability, and Dementia Associated With Self-reported Hearing Problems: A 25-Year Study', *Journal of Gerontology* A Biol Sci Med Sci. 2018 Sep 11;73(10):1383-1389. https://doi.org/10.1093/gerona/glx250

4. '*Another study of 2040 people aged over 50 years . . .*' Ray J, Popli G, Fell G. Association of Cognition and Age-Related Hearing Impairment in the English Longitudinal Study of Ageing (2018), *JAMA Otolaryngology Head and Neck Surgery*, Oct 1;144(10):876-882. https://jamanetwork.com/journals/jamaotolaryngology/fullarticle/2698895

5. '*The current definition of hypertension . . .*' Iqbal AM, Jamal SF, (updated 2022) 'Essential Hypertension', In: StatPearls [Internet]. Treasure Island (FL): StatPearls Publishing, https://www.ncbi.nlm.nih.gov/books/NBK539859/

6. '*The jury is in and we now have more robust evidence . . .*' Sierra C, (2020), 'Hypertension and the Risk of Dementia', *Frontiers in Cardiovascular Medicine*, https://www.frontiersin.org/articles/10.3389/fcvm.2020.00005/full

7. '*A 2017 study found an extra 20 per cent increase in risk of dementia . . .*' McGrath ER, Beiser AS, DeCarli C, Plourde KL, Vasan RS, Greenberg SM, Seshadri S, (2017), 'Blood pressure from mid- to late life and risk of incident dementia', *Neurology*, https://n.neurology.org/content/89/24/2447

8. *'New research has taught us that hypertension disrupts the neurovascular unit . . .'* Hachinski V, Einhäupl K, Ganten D, Alladi S, Brayne C, Stephan BCM, Sweeney MD, Zlokovic B, Iturria-Medina Y, Iadecola C, Nishimura N, Schaffer CB, Whitehead SN, Black SE, Østergaard L, Wardlaw J, Greenberg S, Friberg L, Norrving B, Rowe B, Joanette Y, Hacke W, Kuller L, Dichgans M, Endres M, Khachaturian ZS. (2019) 'Preventing dementia by preventing stroke: The Berlin Manifesto', *Alzheimers & Dementia*, https://alz-journals.onlinelibrary.wiley.com/doi/10.1016/j. jalz.2019.06.001

9. *'Observational studies have shown that treating high blood pressure helps reduce cognitive decline.'* Sierra C, (2020) 'Hypertension and the Risk of Dementia', *Frontiers in Cardiovascular Medicine*, Jan 31;7:5. https://doi.org/10.3389/fcvm.2020.00005

10. *'The Systolic Blood Pressure Intervention Trial (SPRINT) . . .'* Sverre E. Kjeldsen, Krzysztof Narkiewicz, Michel Burnier & Suzanne Oparil (2018) 'Intensive blood pressure lowering prevents mild cognitive impairment and possible dementia and slows development of white matter lesions in brain: the SPRINT Memory and Cognition IN Decreased Hypertension (SPRINT MIND) study,' *Blood Pressure*, 27:5, 247-248, https://doi.org/10.1080/08037051.2018.1507621

11. *'The SPRINT Memory and Cognition in Decreased Hypertension (SPRINT MIND) study took . . .'* Dolui S, Detre JA, Gaussoin SA, et al (2022), 'Association of Intensive vs Standard Blood Pressure Control With Cerebral Blood Flow: Secondary Analysis of the SPRINT MIND Randomized Clinical Trial' JAMA *Neurology*. 79(4):380–389. doi:10.1001/jamaneurol.2022.0074

12. *'The result of their findings, the Berlin Manifesto . . .'* Hachinski V, Einhäupl K, Ganten D, Alladi S, Brayne C, Stephan BCM, Sweeney MD, Zlokovic B, Iturria-Medina Y, Iadecola C, Nishimura N, Schaffer CB, Whitehead SN, Black SE, Østergaard L, Wardlaw J, Greenberg S, Friberg L, Norrving B, Rowe B, Joanette Y, Hacke W, Kuller L, Dichgans M, Endres M, Khachaturian ZS. (2019) 'Preventing dementia by preventing stroke: The Berlin Manifesto', *Alzheimers & Dementia*, https://alz-journals.onlinelibrary.wiley.com/doi/10.1016/j.jalz.2019.06.001

13. *'A meta-analysis of 28 prospective observational studies found that people with type 2 diabetes are 73 per cent more likely to get dementia . . .'* Gudala K, Bansal D, Schifano F, Bhansali A (2013). 'Diabetes mellitus and risk of dementia: A meta-analysis of prospective observational studies', *Journal of Diabetes Investigation*, https://doi.org/10.1111/jdi.12087

14. *'And brain scans of patients with dementia . . .'* Kuehn BM, (2020) 'In Alzheimer Research, Glucose Metabolism Moves to Center Stage', *JAMA*, https://jamanetwork.com/journals/jama/article-abstract/2758712

15. *'. . . with many calling it brain-specific type 3 diabetes.'* de la Monte SM, Wands JR, (2008) 'Alzheimer's Disease is Type 3 Diabetes—Evidence Reviewed', *Journal of Diabetes Science and Technology*, https://journals.sagepub.com/doi/10.1177/193229680800200619

16. *'The authors of a 2017 Cochrane review of seven randomised controlled trials concluded . . .'* Areosa Sastre A, Vernooij RW, González-Colaço Harmand M, Martínez G, (2017) 'Effect of the treatment of Type 2 diabetes mellitus on the development of cognitive impairment and dementia' *Cochrane Database System Review*, https://www.ncbi.nlm.nih.gov/pmc/articles/PMC6481422/.

17. *'In fact, in a couple of trials . . .'* Peters R, Breitner J, James S, Jicha GA, Meyer PF, Richards M, Smith AD, Yassine HN, Abner E, Hainsworth AH, Kehoe PG, Beckett N, Weber C, Anderson C, Anstey KJ, Dodge HH, (2021), 'Dementia risk reduction: why haven't the pharmacological risk reduction trials worked? An in-depth exploration of seven established risk factors', *Alzheimers and Dementia*, https://www.ncbi.nlm.nih.gov/pmc/articles/PMC8655351/

18. *'I was intrigued to read the findings from a Canadian study published in 2020.'* Wu, C-Y, Ouk, M, Wong, YY, et al (2020) 'Relationships between memory decline and the use of metformin or DPP4 inhibitors in people with type 2 diabetes with normal cognition or Alzheimer's disease, and the role ApoE carrier status', *Alzheimer's and Dementia*, https://doi.org/10.1002/alz.12161

19. *'In 2021, a study of data from the UK Biobank cohort based on 500,000 people aged 40–69 years . . .'* (2021) Garfield, V, Farmaki, A-E, Eastwood, SV, et al. 'HbA1c and brain health across the entire glycaemic spectrum', *Diabetes, Obesity and Metabolism*, https://doi.org/10.1111/dom.14321

20. *'Observational data about the link between high cholesterol and dementia . . .'* Reitz C.(2021)

Endnotes

'Dyslipidemia and dementia: current epidemiology, genetic evidence, and mechanisms behind the associations', *Journal of Alzheimers Disease*, https://www.ncbi.nlm.nih.gov/pmc/articles/PMC3689537/

21. *'In 2021, a massive British study of almost two million people . . .'* Masao Iwagami, Nawab Qizilbash, John Gregson, Prof Ian Douglas, Michelle Johnson, Prof Neil Pearce, PhD (2021) 'Blood cholesterol and risk of dementia in more than 1 ·8 million people over two decades: a retrospective cohort study' *The Lancet, Healthy Longevity*, https://doi.org/10.1016/S2666-7568(21)00150-1

22. *'Most specialists agree that high cholesterol will contribute to your overall health . . .'* Laura Perna, Ute Mons Hannah Stocker, Léon Beyer, Konrad Beyreuther, Kira Trares, Bernd Holleczek, Ben Schöttker, Robert Perneczky, Klaus Gerwert, Hermann Brenner, (2022) 'Joint Contributions of markers of Neurodegeneration and Hypercholesterolemia to dementia risk', Medrxiv, https://doi.org/10.1101/2022.01.16.22269370

23. *'Studies have linked high cholesterol with worsening cognition . . .'* Perna L, Mons U, Rujescu D, Kliegel M, Brenner H (2016), 'Apolipoprotein E e4 and Cognitive Function: A Modifiable Association? Results from Two Independent Cohort Studies', *Dementia and Geriatrics Cognitive Disorders*, https://www.karger.com/Article/Abstract/440697#

24. *'To be honest, the data is a bit mixed.'* Peters R, Breitner J, James S, Jicha GA, Meyer PF, Richards M, Smith AD, Yassine HN, Abner E, Hainsworth AH, Kehoe PG, Beckett N, Weber C, Anderson C, Anstey KJ, Dodge HH, (2021) 'Dementia risk reduction: why haven't the pharmacological risk reduction trials worked? An in-depth exploration of seven established risk factors' Alzheimers and Dementia, https://www.ncbi.nlm.nih.gov/pmc/articles/PMC8655351/

25. *'But, ironically, while having high Lp(a) blood levels increases the risk of dementia in APOE e4 carriers . . .'* Röhr F, Bucholtz N, Toepfer S, Norman K, Spira D, Steinhagen-Thiessen E, Lill CM, Bertram L, Demuth I, Buchmann N, Düzel S, (2020) 'Relationship between Lipoprotein (a) and cognitive function - Results from the Berlin Aging Study II', *Scientific Reports*, https://www.ncbi.nlm.nih.gov/pmc/articles/PMC7326928/

26. *'But research tells us that for the people who need them . . .'* https://millionhearts.hhs.gov/learn-prevent/scoop-on-statins.html

27. *'A 2020 US study of 5000 people found a link between dementia risk and higher body mass index . . .'* Anderson, P (2020). 'High BMI in Early Adulthood Linked to Increased Dementia Risk', *Medscape*, https://www.medscape.com/viewarticle/935231#vp_1

28. *'Smokers are at higher risk of dementia than non-smokers . . .'* Choi D, Choi S, Park SM. (2018) 'Effect of smoking cessation on the risk of dementia: a longitudinal study', *Annals of Clinical and Translational Neurology*, https://www.ncbi.nlm.nih.gov/pmc/articles/PMC6186929/

29. *'In one study of 50,000 men aged older than 60 years . . .'* Choi D, Choi S, Park SM. (2018) 'Effect of smoking cessation on the risk of dementia: a longitudinal study', *Annals of Clinical and Translational Neurology*, https://www.ncbi.nlm.nih.gov/pmc/articles/PMC6186929/

30. *'One study of women aged 55–64 years . . .'* Pan X, Luo Y, Roberts AR. (2018) 'Secondhand Smoke and Women's Cognitive Function in China', American Journal of Epidemiology, https://doi.org/10.1093/aje/kwx377

31. *'One looked at women with an average age of 82 . . .'* Yaffe K, Laffan AM, Harrison SL, Redline S, Spira AP, Ensrud KE, Ancoli-Israel S, Stone KL, (2011). 'Sleep-disordered breathing, hypoxia, and risk of mild cognitive impairment and dementia in older women', *JAMA*. https://www.ncbi.nlm.nih.gov/pmc/articles/PMC3600944/

32. *'A British study found that many people in clinics for frailty . . .'* Eef Hogervorst, Felicia Huppert, Fiona E. Matthews, Carol Brayne, (2008). 'Thyroid function and cognitive decline in the MRC Cognitive Function and Ageing Study' *Psychoneuroendocrinology*, Vol 33, Issue 7, https://doi.org/10.1016/j.psyneuen.2008.05.008

33. *'A massive 2021 Danish study found anywhere from 10–20 per cent increase risk . . .'* Thvilum M, Brandt F, Lillevang-Johansen M, Folkestad L, Brix TH, Hegedüs L. (2021) 'Increased risk of dementia in hypothyroidism: A Danish nationwide register-based study'. *Clinical Endocrinology*, https://onlinelibrary.wiley.com/doi/10.1111/cen.14424

34. *'Periodontitis gives you more than halitosis and tooth loss . . .'* Rocha FG, Berges A, Sedra A, Ghods S, Kapoor N, Pill L, Davey ME, Fairman J and Gibson FC III, (2021), 'A Porphyromonas gingivalis Capsule-Conjugate Vaccine Protects From Experimental Oral Bone Loss', *Frontiers in Oral Health* https://doi.org/10.3389/froh.2021.686402

35. *'A recent US study found that the same bacteria that cause gum disease . . .'* https://www.nia.nih.gov/news/large-study-links-gum-disease-dementia

36. *'Many of these bacteria produce toxic proteins . . .'* Demmer RT, Norby FL, Lakshminarayan K, Walker KA, Pankow JS, Folsom AR, Mosley T, Beck J, Lutsey PL. (2020) 'Periodontal disease and incident dementia: The Atherosclerosis Risk in Communities Study (ARIC)', *Neurology*, https://www.ncbi.nlm.nih.gov/pmc/articles/PMC7713724/

37. *'The study looked at data from the National Health and Nutrition Examination Survey (NHANES) . .'* Centers for Disease Control and Prevention, https://www.cdc.gov/nchs/nhanes/index.htm

38. *'Another large US study published in 2020 found that having gum disease gave people a 20 per cent higher chance of developing . . .'* Demmer RT, Norby FL, Lakshminarayan K, Walker KA, Pankow JS, Folsom AR, Mosley T, Beck J, Lutsey PL. (2020) 'Periodontal disease and incident dementia: The Atherosclerosis Risk in Communities Study (ARIC)'. *Neurology.* https://www.ncbi.nlm.nih.gov/pmc/articles/PMC7713724/

39. *'So, research for a vaccine against the P. Gingivalis bacteria is underway.'* Rocha FG, Berges A, Sedra A, Ghods S, Kapoor N, Pill L, Davey ME, Fairman J and Gibson FC III (2021) 'A Porphyromonas gingivalis Capsule-Conjugate Vaccine Protects From Experimental Oral Bone Loss'. Frontiers in Oral Health, https://doi.org/10.3389/froh.2021.686402

49. *'Replace your toothbrush when the bristles start splaying . . .'*, Van Leeuwen MPC, Van der Weijden FA, Slot DE, Rosema MAM. (2019) 'Toothbrush wear in relation to toothbrushing effectiveness'. *International Journal of Dental Hygiene*

50. *'. . . or go for an electric toothbrush . . .'* Bahammam S, Chen CY, Ishida Y, Hayashi A, Ikeda Y, Ishii H, Kim DM, Nagai S. (2021) 'Electric and Manual Oral Hygiene Routines Affect Plaque Index Score Differently'. *International Journal Environmental Research and Public Health*, https://www.mdpi.com/1660-4601/18/24/13123

51. *'A UK study comparing before and after MRI scans of patients with COVID-19 found that parts of the brain can be affected 20 weeks . . .'* Douaud, G., Lee, S., Alfaro-Almagro, F. et a, (2022). 'SARS-CoV-2 is associated with changes in brain structure in UK Biobank', *Nature*, https://doi.org/10.1038/s41586-022-04569-5

Chapter 8

1. *'The results vary, but, on the whole, late-life depression gives you . . .'* Byers AL, Yaffe K. (2011) 'Depression and risk of developing dementia'. *Nature Reviews Neurology*, https://doi.org/10.1038/nrneurol.2011.60

2. *'Indeed, a 2004 study seemed to support this . . .'* Modrego PJ, Ferrández J. (2004), 'Depression in Patients With Mild Cognitive Impairment Increases the Risk of Developing Dementia of Alzheimer Type: A Prospective Cohort Study', *Archives of Neurology.*

3. *'Certainly MRI studies show shrinkage of parts of the brain . . .'* Hurley LL, Tizabi Y. (2013) 'Neuroinflammation, neurodegeneration, and depression', *Neurotoxicity Research*, https://link.springer.com/article/10.1007/s12640-012-9348-1

4. *'We know that antidepressant medication is not just a symptom reliever . . .'* (2103), Kim HJ, Kim W, Kong SY. Antidepressants for neuro-regeneration: from depression to Alzheimer's disease. *Archives of Pharmacal Research*, https://link.springer.com/article/10.1007/s12272-013-0238-8

5. *'It's thought that exercise causes the blood vessels to open up . . .'* Sharma A, Madaan V, Petty FD. (2006) 'Exercise for mental health', Primary Care Companion, *Journal of Clinical Psychiatry*, https://pubmed.ncbi.nlm.nih.gov/16862239/

6. *'Aerobic exercises, including jogging, swimming, cycling, walking, gardening and dancing . . .'* Guszkowska M. Wpływ ćwiczeń fizycznych na poziom leku i depresji oraz stany nastroju, (2004) [Effects of exercise on anxiety, depression and mood]. *Psychiatria polska*, https://pubmed.ncbi.nlm.nih.gov/15518309/

7. *'The sounds of nature . . .'* Alvarsson JJ, Wiens S, Nilsson ME. (2010) 'Stress recovery during

Endnotes

exposure to nature sound and environmental noise,' *International Journal of Environmental Research in Public Health*, https://www.mdpi.com/1660-4601/7/3/1036

8. *'Group walks in nature . . .'* Marselle, Melissa & Irvine, Katherine & Warber, Sara. (2014). 'Examining Group Walks in Nature and Multiple Aspects of Well-Being: A Large-Scale Study', *Ecopsychology*, https://www.liebertpub.com/doi/abs/10.1089/eco.2014.0027

9. *'Even gardening has been shown . . .'* Van Den Berg AE, Custers MHG, (2011) 'Gardening Promotes Neuroendocrine and Affective Restoration from Stress'. *Journal of Health Psychology*, https://journals.sagepub.com/doi/abs/10.1177/1359105310365577

10. *'The worse your diet, the higher the risk . . .'* Hussein N Yassine (2022) 'Nutrition state of science and dementia prevention: recommendations of the Nutrition for Dementia Prevention Working Group', *The Lancet Healthy Longevity*, https://doi.org/10.1016/S2666-7568(22)00120-9

11. *'But it has good evidence as a treatment for depression.'* Pim Cuijpers, Eirini Karyotaki, Leonore de Wit & David D. Ebert (2020) 'The effects of fifteen evidence-supported therapies for adult depression: A meta-analytic review', *Psychotherapy Research*, https://doi.org/10.1080/10503307.2019.1649732

12. *'The evidence is mounting that bypassing the personal therapist and opting for an app is a great, and definitely cheaper, option!'* Malhi G, Bell E, Bassett D, Boyce P, Bryant R, Hazell P, Hopwood M, Lyndon B, Mulder R, Porter R, Singh A, Murray G. (2020) 'The 2020 Royal Australian and New Zealand College of Psychiatrists clinical practice guidelines for mood disorders', *Australian & New Zealand Journal of Psychiatry* , https://www.ranzcp.org/files/resources/college_statements/clinician/cpg/mood-disorders-cpg-2020.aspx

13. *'In 2018, a huge meta-analysis of trials was published the prestigious medical journal . . .'* Cipriani, Andrea et al, (2018). 'Comparative efficacy and acceptability of 21 antidepressant drugs for the acute treatment of adults with major depressive disorder: a systematic review and network meta-analysis', *The Lancet*, https://doi.org/10.1016/S0140-6736(17)32802-7

14. *'Transcranial magnetic stimulation'.* https://www.blackdoginstitute.org.au/resources-support/depression/treatment/

15. *'A recent review of studies found no randomised controlled trials at all.'* Haller H, Anheyer D, Cramer H, Dobos G. (2019) 'Complementary therapies for clinical depression: an overview of systematic reviews', *BMJ Open*, https://www.ncbi.nlm.nih.gov/pmc/articles/PMC6686993/

16. *'Studies of aromatherapy . . .'* Ball EL, Owen-Booth B, Gray A, Shenkin SD, Hewitt J, McCleery J, (2020) 'Aromatherapy for dementia', *Cochrane Database System Review*, https://www.ncbi.nlm.nih.gov/pmc/articles/PMC7437395/

17. *'. . . in a recent review of studies to benefit people . . .'* Watt JA, Goodarzi Z, Veroniki AA, Nincic V, Khan PA, Ghassemi M, Lai Y, Treister V, Thompson Y, Schneider R, Tricco AC, Straus SE. (2021) 'Comparative efficacy of interventions for reducing symptoms of depression in people with dementia: systematic review and network meta-analysis'. *BMJ*. https://www.bmj.com/content/372/bmj.n532

18. *'A 2017 meta-analysis of six trials of curcumin for depression . . .'* 'Clinical Use of Curcumin in Depression: A Meta-Analysis' Ng, Qin Xiang et al. (2017) *Journal of the American Medical Directors Association*, Vol 18, https://www.jamda.com/article/S1525-8610(16)30675-2/fulltext

19. *'Light therapy'.* Haller H, Anheyer D, Cramer H, Dobos G. (2019) 'Complementary therapies for clinical depression: an overview of systematic reviews', BMJ Open https://www.ncbi.nlm.nih.gov/pmc/articles/PMC6686993/

20. *'For patients with seasonal depression . . .'* Pjrek E, Friedrich ME, Cambioli L, Dold M, Jäger F, Komorowski A, Lanzenberger R, Kasper S, Winkler D. (2020) 'The Efficacy of Light Therapy in the Treatment of Seasonal Affective Disorder: A Meta-Analysis of Randomized Controlled Trials', *Psychotherapy and Psychosomatics*. https://www.karger.com/Article/Abstract/502891

21. *'A high-quality Cochrane review meta-analysed 49 studies . . .'* Smith CA, Armour M, Lee MS, Wang LQ, Hay PJ. (2018) 'Acupuncture for depression', *Cochrane Database of Systematic Reviews*, https://www.cochranelibrary.com/cdsr/doi/10.1002/14651858.CD004046.pub4/full

22. *'Another Cochrane review, this time from 2008 . . .'* Linde K, Berner M, Kriston L, (2008) 'St John's

wort for major depression', *Cochrane Database of Systematic Reviews*, https://doi.org/10.1002/14651858.CD000448.pub3

23. *'Once again, we have a Cochrane review to draw on . . .'* Galizia I, Oldani L, Macritchie K, Amari E, Dougall D, Jones TN, Lam RW, Massei GJ, Yatham LN, Young AH, (2016) 'S-adenosyl methionine (SAMe) for depression in adults', *Cochrane Database of Systematic Reviews*, https://doi.org/10.1002/14651858.CD011286.pub2

24. *'A 2015 Cochrane review of 25 studies including 1400 people . . .'* Appleton KM, Sallis HM, Perry R, Ness AR, Churchill R. (2015) 'Omega-3 fatty acids for depression in adults', *Cochrane Database of Systematic Reviews* , https://doi.org/10.1002/14651858.CD004692.pub4

25. *'There is some evidence from tiny trials that massage may decrease . . .'* Rapaport MH, Schettler PJ, Larson ER, Carroll D, Sharenko M, Nettles J, Kinkead B. (2018) 'Massage Therapy for Psychiatric Disorders. *Focus*, American Psychiatric Publication, https://focus.psychiatryonline.org/doi/10.1176/appi.focus.20170043

26. *'For vitamin B6 supplements, a review of just two studies . . .'* Anna-leila Williams, Anne Cotter, Alyse Sabina, Christine Girard, Jonathan Goodman, David L Katz, (2005) 'The role for vitamin B-6 as treatment for depression: a systematic review', *Family Practice*, Vol 22, https://doi.org/10.1093/fampra/cmi040

27. *'For folic acid (AKA vitamin B9) supplements . . .'* Taylor MJ, Carney SM, Geddes J, Goodwin G. (2003) 'Folate for depressive disorders'. *Cochrane Database of Systematic Reviews*, https://doi.org/10.1002/14651858.CD003390

28. *'A 2014 meta-analysis of vitamin D supplements for depression . . .'* Shaffer, Jonathan A. PhD, MS; Edmondson, Donald PhD, MPH; Wasson, Lauren Taggart MD, MPH; Falzon, Louise PGDipInf; Homma, Kirsten BA; Ezeokoli, Nchedcochukwu; Li, Peter BA; Davidson, Karina W. PhD. (2014) 'Vitamin D Supplementation for Depressive Symptoms: A Systematic Review and Meta-Analysis of Randomized Controlled Trials', *Psychosomatic Medicine*, https://journals.lww.com/psychosomaticmedicine/Abstract/2014/04000/Vitamin_D_Supplementation_for_Depressive_Symptoms_.9.aspx

29. *'. . . a "window of vulnerability". . .'* Pauline M. Maki, Susan G. Kornstein, Hadine Joffe, Joyce T. Bromberger, Ellen W. Freeman, Geena Athappilly, William V. Bobo, Leah H. Rubin, Hristina K. Koleva, Lee S. Cohen, Claudio N. Soares, and on behalf of the Board of Trustees for The North American Menopause Society (NAMS) and the Women and Mood Disorders Task Force of the National Network of Depression Centers, (2019), 'Guidelines for the Evaluation and Treatment of Perimenopausal Depression: Summary and Recommendations', *Journal of Women's Health*, http://doi.org/10.1089/jwh.2018.27099.mensocrec

30. *'For peri women – you are between . . .'* Bromberger JT, Kravitz HM, Chang YF, Cyranowski JM, Brown C, Matthews KA. (2011) 'Major depression during and after the menopausal transition: Study of Women's Health Across the Nation (SWAN)'. *Psychological Medicine*. doi:10.1017/S003329171100016X

31. *'If you have ever had a battle with depression . . .'* Maki, Pauline (2021) 'Identifying and treating perimenopausal depression', https://www.youtube.com/watch?v=AmSV5Yj3kPo

32. *'Depression in perimenopause often has distinct characteristics . . .'* Pauline M. Maki, Susan G. Kornstein, Hadine Joffe, Joyce T. Bromberger, Ellen W. Freeman, Geena Athappilly, William V. Bobo, Leah H. Rubin, Hristina K. Koleva, Lee S. Cohen, Claudio N. Soares, and on behalf of the Board of Trustees for The North American Menopause Society (NAMS) and the Women and Mood Disorders Task Force of the National Network of Depression Centers, (2019), 'Guidelines for the Evaluation and Treatment of Perimenopausal Depression: Summary and Recommendations', *Journal of Women's Health*, http://doi.org/10.1089/jwh.2018.27099.mensocrec

33. *'There is some evidence that HRT has an effect . . .'* Gava G, Orsili I, Alvisi S, Mancini I, Seracchioli R, Meriggiola MC. (2019) 'Cognition, Mood and Sleep in Menopausal Transition: The Role of Menopause Hormone Therapy', *Medicina* https://www.ncbi.nlm.nih.gov/pmc/articles/PMC6843314/

Endnotes

34. *'Research published in 2018 from the University of North Carolina School...'* Williams, Jamie, UNS Health and UNC School of Medicine, (2018), https://news.unchealthcare.org/2018/01/hormone-therapy-could-effectively-prevent-depression-for-some-women-in-the-menopause-transition/

35. *'Professor Pauline Maki suggested in a webinar to the International Menopause Society that certain women...'* Maki, Pauline (2021) 'Identifying and treating perimenopausal depression', https://www.youtube.com/watch?v=AmSV5Yj3kPo

36. *'US data suggests anxiety is the most common mental illness in the US...'* Anxiety and Depression Association of America, https://adaa.org/understanding-anxiety/facts-statistics

37. *'And that number only went up in the pandemic.'* COVID-19 Mental Disorders Collaborators. (2021) Global prevalence and burden of depressive and anxiety disorders in 204 countries and territories in 2020 due to the COVID-19 pandemic', *The Lancet*, https://www.thelancet.com/journals/lancet/article/PIIS0140-6736(21)02143-7/fulltext

38. *'A meta-analysis of six studies of older adults found that those with anxiety ...'* Santabárbara J, Lipnicki DM, Olaya B, Villagrasa B, Bueno-Notivol J, Nuez L, López-Antón R, Gracia-García P. (2020) 'Does Anxiety Increase the Risk of All-Cause Dementia? An Updated Meta-Analysis of Prospective Cohort Studies', *Journal of Clinical Medicine*, https://www.mdpi.com/2077-0383/9/6/1791

39. *'Then in 2021 a new US study was published ...'* Ahn S, Mathiason MA, Yu F. (2021) 'Longitudinal Cognitive Profiles by Anxiety and Depressive Symptoms in American Older Adults With Subjective Cognitive Decline'. *Journal of Nursing Scholarship*, https://sigmapubs.onlinelibrary.wiley.com/doi/10.1111/jnu.12692

40. *'A 2018 meta-analysis of four studies comprising almost 30,000 people ...'* Gimson A, Schlosser M, Huntley JD, Marchant NL, (2018), 'Support for midlife anxiety diagnosis as an independent risk factor for dementia: a systematic review'. *BMJ Open*, https://bmjopen.bmj.com/content/8/4/e019399

41. *'The Australian Imaging, Biomarker & Lifestyle Flagship Study of Ageing (AIBL) is the largest study of its kind in Australia.'* https://aibl.csiro.au

42. *'The results have started coming in from various studies from this major research ...'* Pink, A, Krell-Roesch, J, Syrjanen, JA, et al. (2021) 'A longitudinal investigation of Aβ, anxiety, depression, and mild cognitive impairment'. *Alzheimer's and Dementia*, https://doi.org/10.1002/alz.12504

43. *'... a study based on the AIBL data found...'* Holmes SE, Esterlis I, Mazure CM, Lim YY, Ames D, Rainey-Smith S, Fowler C, Ellis K, Martins RN, Salvado O, Doré V, Villemagne VL, Rowe CC, Laws SM, Masters CL, Pietrzak RH, Maruff P; (2018) 'Australian Imaging, Biomarkers and Lifestyle Research Group. Trajectories of depressive and anxiety symptoms in older adults: a 6-year prospective cohort study', *International Journal of Geriatric Psychiatry*, https://onlinelibrary.wiley.com/doi/10.1002/gps.4761

44. *'In 2022, a study was published in the journal Neurology ...'* Joel Salinas, Alexa S. Beiser, Jasmeet K. Samra, AdrienneO'Donnell, Charles S. DeCarli, Mitzi M. Gonzales, Hugo J. Aparicio, Sudha Seshadri (2022) 'Association of Loneliness With 10-Year Dementia Risk and Early Markers of Vulnerability for Neurocognitive Decline', *Neurology*, https://n.neurology.org/content/98/13/e1337

45. *'This followed another study of 60,000 people published just a month earlier ...'* Golaszewski NM, LaCroix AZ, Godino JG, et al. (2021) 'Evaluation of Social Isolation, Loneliness, and Cardiovascular Disease Among Older Women in the US' *JAMA Network Open*, https://jamanetwork.com/journals/jamanetworkopen/fullarticle/2788582

Chapter 9

1. *'I was alarmed by a 2017 meta-analysis of 27 studies that found sleep problems ...'* Omonigho M. Bubu, MD, MPH, Michael Brannick, PhD, James Mortimer, PhD, Ogie Umasabor-Bubu, MD MPH, Yuri V. Sebastião, MPH, Yi Wen, MS, Skai Schwartz, PhD, Amy R. Borenstein, PhD, Yougui Wu, PhD, David Morgan, PhD, William M. Anderson, MD. (2017) 'Sleep, Cognitive impairment, and Alzheimer's disease: A Systematic Review and Meta-Analysis', *Sleep*, Vol 40 https://academic.oup.com/sleep/article/40/1/zsw032/2661823

2. *'... we know that there is a 'switch' for sleep – the ventrolateral preoptic nucleus (VLPO) ...'* Gaus SE, Strecker RE, Tate BA, Parker RA, Saper CB. (2002) 'Ventrolateral preoptic nucleus contains sleep-active, galaninergic neurons in multiple mammalian species', *Neuroscience*, https://pubmed.ncbi.nlm.nih.gov/12401341/

3. *'Normal sleep goes through rhythmic sleep cycles ...'* Institute for Quality and Efficiency in Health Care (IQWiG) 2013 [Updated 2016] 'What is "normal" sleep?' https://www.ncbi.nlm.nih.gov/books/NBK279322/

4. *'If you look at total sleep time, it decreases year on year ...'* Lavoie, C.J., Zeidler, M.R. & Martin, J.L. (2018) 'Sleep and aging', Sleep Science Practice Vol 2, https://doi.org/10.1186/s41606-018-0021-3

5. *'Unfortunately, the glymphatic system degrades with age.'* Nedergaard M, Steven Goldman S, (2020), 'Glymphatic failure as a final common pathway to dementia', *Science*, https://doi.org/10.1126/science.abb8739

6. *'This part of the brain sees a depletion in the number of cells ...'* Elda Arrigoni, Patrick M. Fuller, Chapter 4 'An Overview of Sleep: Physiology and Neuroanatomy', *Therapy in Sleep Medicine*, https://doi.org/10.1016/B978-1-4377-1703-7.10004-0

7. *'Plus, it seems the connections within this part of the brain become more fragmented ...'* Singletary KG, Naidoo N. (2011) 'Disease and Degeneration of Aging Neural Systems that Integrate Sleep Drive and Circadian Oscillations', Frontiers in Neurology, https://www.ncbi.nlm.nih.gov/pmc/articles/PMC3199684/

8. *'It is not just our sleep but our daily ...'* The Florey Institute of Neuroscience and Mental Health, https://florey.edu.au/science-research/research-projects/food-entrainment-of-circadian-rhythms

9. *'This timing of the cycle is controlled by a kind of circadian pacemaker ...'* Boyce P, Barriball E. (2010) 'Circadian rhythms and depression', https://www.racgp.org.au

10. *'Your melatonin levels peak at 3 or 4 a.m. ...'* Atul Khullar, MD, MSc (2012) 'The Role of Melatonin in the Circadian Rhythm Sleep-Wake Cycle' *Psychiatric Times*, Vol 29, https://www.psychiatrictimes.com/view/role-melatonin-circadian-rhythm-sleep-wake-cycle

11. *'Exactly how melatonin works ...'* Rajaratnam SM, Middleton B, Stone BM, Arendt J, Dijk DJ, (2004). 'Melatonin advances the circadian timing of EEG sleep and directly facilitates sleep without altering its duration in extended sleep opportunities in humans', *Journal of Physiology*, https://physoc.onlinelibrary.wiley.com/doi/10.1113/jphysiol.2004.073742

12. *'... it's been proven to be a powerful antioxidant ...'* Bubenik GA, Konturek SJ (2011), 'Melatonin and aging: prospects for human treatment', *Journal of Physiology and Pharmacology*, https://pubmed.ncbi.nlm.nih.gov/21451205/

13. *'Natural melatonin levels increase from birth ...'* Shukla M, Govitrapong P, Boontem P, Reiter RJ, Satayavivad J. (2017) 'Mechanisms of Melatonin in Alleviating Alzheimer's Disease', *Current Neuropharmacology*, https://www.eurekaselect.com/article/82252

14. *'Certainly, some studies suggest melatonin directly prevents the build-up of amyloid in the brain ...'* Shukla M, Govitrapong P, Boontem P, Reiter RJ, Satayavivad J. (2017) 'Mechanisms of Melatonin in Alleviating Alzheimer's Disease', *Current Neuropharmacology*, https://www.eurekaselect.com/article/82252

15. *'And in other studies melatonin ...'* Shukla M, Govitrapong P, Boontem P, Reiter RJ, Satayavivad J. (2017) 'Mechanisms of Melatonin in Alleviating Alzheimer's Disease', *Current Neuropharmacology*, https://www.eurekaselect.com/article/82252

16. *'Another key hormone in regulating sleep is orexin, which is sometimes called hypocretin.'* Hickie, I.B., Naismith, S.L., Robillard, R. et al (2013). 'Manipulating the sleep-wake cycle and circadian rhythms to improve clinical management of major depression'. *BMC Medicine*, https://doi.org/10.1186/1741-7015-11-79

17. *'... have between 85 and 90 per cent fewer orexin producing neurons.'* Thannickal TC, Moore RY, Nienhuis R, Ramanathan L, Gulyani S, Aldrich M, Cornford M, Siegel JM. (2000) 'Reduced number of hypocretin neurons in human narcolepsy', *Neuron*. https://pubmed.ncbi.nlm.nih.gov/11055430/

Endnotes

18. *'Recent studies have confirmed links between higher orexin levels and binge eating, pain, addiction and stress.'* Grafe LA, Bhatnagar S. (2018) 'Orexins and stress'. *Frontiers in Neuroendocrinology*. https://doi. org/10.1016/j.yfrne.2018.06.003

19. *'Studies have shown that anxiety turbo charges your orexin levels . . .'* Johnson, Phillip (2017) 'Hypothalamic Orexin Role in Menopause-Associated Hot Flashes and Mood/Sleep Disruption', https://grantome.com/grant/NIH/K01-AG044466-01A1

20. *'Typically, the low point for cortisol levels is somewhere around midnight.'* Hirotsu C, Tufik S, Andersen ML. (2015) 'Interactions between sleep, stress, and metabolism: From physiological to pathological conditions', *Sleep Science*, https://www.ncbi.nlm.nih.gov/pmc/articles/PMC4688585/

21. *'But cortisol levels start to increase in the evening . . .'* Van Cauter E, Leproult R, Plat L (2000). 'Age-related changes in slow wave sleep and REM sleep and relationship with growth hormone and cortisol levels in healthy men'. *JAMA* https://jamanetwork.com/journals/jama/fullarticle/192981

22. *'Perimenopause is another time when your cortisol levels go up . . .'* Woods NF, Mitchell ES, Smith-Dijulio K. (2009) 'Cortisol levels during the menopausal transition and early postmenopause: observations from the Seattle Midlife Women's Health Study', *Menopause*. https://www.ncbi. nlm.nih.gov/pmc/articles/PMC2749064/

23. *'So even young women with natural cycles tend to have more disrupted sleep before their period starts . . .'* Bezerra AG, Andersen ML, Pires GN, Tufik S, Hachul H. 'Effects of hormonal contraceptives on sleep – A possible treatment for insomnia in premenopausal women', *Sleep Science*, https://www.ncbi. nlm.nih.gov/pmc/articles/PMC6201525/.

24. *'At a cellular level, sleep is critical for the elimination of waste . . .'* Green TRF, Ortiz JB, Wonnacott S, Williams RJ and Rowe RK (2020) 'The Bidirectional Relationship Between Sleep and Inflammation Links Traumatic Brain Injury and Alzheimer's Disease', *Frontiers in Neuroscience*, https:// www.frontiersin.org/articles/10.3389/fnins.2020.00894/full

25. *'. . . as well as neuroplasticity . . .'* Puentes-Mestril C, Aton SJ. (2017) 'Linking Network Activity to Synaptic Plasticity during Sleep: Hypotheses and Recent Data', *Frontiers in Neural Circuits*, https://doi.org/10.3389/fncir.2017.00061

26. *'Sleep is the time when we consolidate our memories.'* Davidson P, Jönsson P, Carlsson I, Pace-Schott E (2021), 'Does Sleep Selectively Strengthen Certain Memories Over Others Based on Emotion and Perceived Future Relevance?' *Natural Science Sleep*, https://doi.org/10.2147/NSS.S286701

27. *'Sleep deprivation impairs performance on tasks that test cognitive ability . . .'* Seugnet L, Dissel S, Thimgan M, Cao L, Shaw PJ (2017). 'Identification of Genes that Maintain Behavioral and Structural Plasticity during Sleep Loss', *Frontiers in Neural Circuits*, https://doi.org/10.3389/fncir.2017.00079

28. *'Studies in mice models shows that sleep . . .'* Bellesi M, de Vivo L, Chini M, Gilli F, Tononi G, Cirelli C. (2017) 'Sleep Loss Promotes Astrocytic Phagocytosis and Microglial Activation in Mouse Cerebral Cortex', *Journal of Neuroscience*. https://pubmed.ncbi.nlm.nih.gov/28539349/

29. *'Beyond the brain, sleep kickstarts the immune system.'* Besedovsky L, Lange T, Haack M. (2019) 'The Sleep-Immune Crosstalk in Health and Disease'. *Physiological Reviews*, https://www.ncbi.nlm. nih.gov/pmc/articles/PMC6689741/

30. *'After just one bad night's sleep, nerve fibres from your sympathetic nervous system . . .'* Irwin MR, Opp MR (2017), 'Sleep Health: Reciprocal Regulation of Sleep and Innate Immunity, *Neuropsychopharmacology*, https://www.ncbi.nlm.nih.gov/pmc/articles/PMC5143488/

31. *'. . . 70 per cent of people with diagnosed cognitive impairment or dementia have some sort of sleep disturbances.'* Wennberg AMV, Wu MN, Rosenberg PB, Spira AP. Sleep Disturbance, Cognitive Decline, and Dementia: A Review', *Seminars in Neurology*, https://www.ncbi.nlm.nih.gov/pmc/articles/PMC5910033/

32. *'I already mentioned the 2017 meta-analysis of 27 studies covering almost 70,000 people . . .'* Omonigho M. Bubu, MD, MPH, Michael Brannick, PhD, James Mortimer, PhD, Ogie Umasabor-Bubu, MD MPH, Yuri V. Sebastião, MPH, Yi Wen, MS, Skai Schwartz, PhD, Amy R. Borenstein, PhD, Yougui Wu, PhD, David Morgan, PhD, William M. Anderson, MD. (2017) 'Sleep, Cognitive impairment,

and Alzheimer's disease: A Systematic Review and Meta-Analysis', *Sleep*, Vol 40, https://doi.org/10.1093/sleep/zsw032

33. *'From a Whitehall study published in 2021 . . .'* Sabia, S., Fayosse, A., Dumurgier, J. et al (2021). 'Association of sleep duration in middle and old age with incidence of dementia', *Nature Communications*, https://doi.org/10.1038/s41467-021-22354-2

34. *'The current thinking is that the relationship between lack of sleep is bidirectional.'* Wennberg AMV, Wu MN, Rosenberg PB, Spira AP., (2017) 'Sleep Disturbance, Cognitive Decline, and Dementia: A Review', *Seminars in Neurology,* https://www.ncbi.nlm.nih.gov/pmc/articles/PMC5910033/

35. *'One study of almost 28,000 people in China and the UK, reported in 2020 . . .'* Ma Y, Liang L, Zheng F, Shi L, Zhong B, Xie W (2020). 'Association Between Sleep Duration and Cognitive Decline' *JAMA Network Open.* https://www.ncbi.nlm.nih.gov/pmc/articles/PMC7506513/

36. *'There was a small Korean study published in 2018 . . .'* Suh, S.W., Han, J.W., Lee, J.R., Byun, S., Kwon, S.J., Oh, S.H., Lee, K.H., Han, G., Hong, J.W., Kwak, K.P., Kim, B.-J., Kim, S.G., Kim, J.L., Kim, T.H., Ryu, S.-H., Moon, S.W., Park, J.H., Seo, J., Youn, J.C., Lee, D.Y., Lee, D.W., Lee, S.B., Lee, J.J., Jhoo, J.H. and Kim, K.W. (2018), 'Sleep and cognitive decline: A prospective non-demented elderly cohort study', *Annals of Neurology*, https://doi.org/10.1002/ana.25166

37. *'A 2016 German study of 800 people found that those with broken sleep . . .'* ohar H, Kawan R, Emeny RT, Ladwig KH. (2016) 'Impaired Sleep Predicts Cognitive Decline in Old People: Findings from the Prospective KORA Age Study', *Sleep*, https://www.ncbi.nlm.nih.gov/pmc/articles/PMC4678344/

38. *'Studies suggest that between 30 and 40 per cent of insomnia is in your genes (up to 250 of them have been identified so far).'* Byrne EM. (2019) 'The relationship between insomnia and complex diseases-insights from genetic data', *Genome Medicine.* https://pubmed.ncbi.nlm.nih.gov/31466529/

39. *'Many experts assert that that there is probably a "bidirectional link" between disturbed sleep and dementia . . .'* Wennberg AMV, Wu MN, Rosenberg PB, Spira AP., (2017) 'Sleep Disturbance, Cognitive Decline, and Dementia: A Review', *Seminars in Neurology,* https://www.ncbi.nlm.nih.gov/pmc/articles/PMC5910033/

40. *'We know from research that the later you get your face . . .'* Quante M, Mariani S, Weng J, Marinac CR, Kaplan ER, Rueschman M, Mitchell JA, James P, Hipp JA, Cespedes Feliciano EM, Wang R, Redline S. (2019) 'Zeitgebers and their association with rest-activity patterns', *Chronobiology International.* https://www.ncbi.nlm.nih.gov/pmc/articles/PMC6492024/

41. *'But, for this shutdown to happen you need a light intensity of at least 1500 lux (brighter than standard artificial lighting).'* Boyce P, Barriball E. (2010) 'Circadian rhythms and depression', https://www.racgp.org.au

42. *'. . . but exercise can be used as a zeitgeber to enhance your sleep if you exercise at a regular time every day.'* Lewis P, Korf HW, Kuffer L, Groß JV, Erren TC. (2018) 'Exercise time cues (zeitgebers) for human circadian systems can foster health and improve performance: a systematic review', *BMJ Open Sport Exercise Medicine.* https://www.ncbi.nlm.nih.gov/pmc/articles/PMC6330200/

43. *'In a 2021 study from Hong Kong of older adults . . .'* Siu PM, Yu AP, Tam BT, et al (2021). 'Effects of Tai Chi or Exercise on Sleep in Older Adults With Insomnia: A Randomized Clinical Trial', *JAMA Network Open,* https://jamanetwork.com/journals/jamanetworkopen/fullarticle/2776441

44. *'An interesting Israeli study showed that people who followed a regular daily routine . . .'* Zisberg A, Gur-Yaish N, Shochat T.(2010) 'Contribution of routine to sleep quality in community elderly', *Sleep*, https://www.ncbi.nlm.nih.gov/pmc/articles/PMC2849790/

45. *'There is some evidence for yoga, abdominal breathing and progressive muscle relaxation too.'* Maness DL, Khan M. (2015) 'Nonpharmacologic Management of Chronic Insomnia', *American Family Physician*, https://pubmed.ncbi.nlm.nih.gov/26760592/

46. *'In 2019, a meta-analysis of 13 trials . . .'* Davidson JR, Dickson C, Han H (2019). 'Cognitive behavioural treatment for insomnia in primary care: a systematic review of sleep outcomes', *British Journal of General Practitioners* https://www.ncbi.nlm.nih.gov/pmc/articles/PMC6663098/

Endnotes

47. *'The data is less compelling for its ability . . .'* Hartmann E (1982-1983) 'Effects of L-tryptophan on sleepiness and on sleep', *Journal of Psychiatric Research.* https://doi.org/10.1016/0022-3956(82)90012-7

48. *'Although the effect of tryptophan on sleep has been studied only over the short term . . .'* Young SN (2003). 'Is tryptophan a natural hypnotic?' *Journal of Psychiatry and Neuroscience,* https://www.ncbi.nlm.nih.gov/pmc/issues/5152/

49. *'A 2021 meta-analysis of five studies . . .'* Cheah KL, Norhayati MN, Husniati Yaacob L, Abdul Rahman R (2021). 'Effect of Ashwagandha (Withania somnifera) extract on sleep: A systematic review and meta-analysis', *Plos one,* https://www.ncbi.nlm.nih.gov/pmc/articles/PMC8462692/

50. *'Studies show that around 40 per cent of adults with insomnia . . .'* Bent S, Padula A, Moore D, Patterson M, Mehling W (2006). 'Valerian for sleep: a systematic review and meta-analysis', *American Journal of Medicine,* https://www.ncbi.nlm.nih.gov/pmc/articles/PMC4394901/

51. *'The data we have suggests that higher doses are safe . . .'* Menczel Schrire Z, Phillips CL, Chapman JL, Duffy SL, Wong G, D'Rozario AL, Comas M, Raisin I, Saini B, Gordon CJ, McKinnon AC, Naismith SL, Marshall NS, Grunstein RR, Hoyos CM., (2022), 'Safety of higher doses of melatonin in adults: A systematic review and meta-analysis', *Journal of Pineal Research,* https://pubmed.ncbi.nlm.nih.gov/34923676/ 2022

52. *'Diphenhydramine is not recommended for the elderly . . .'* Eng, M. (2008) 'Potentially Inappropriate OTC Medications in Older Adults', *US Pharmacist.* US Pharm. 2008;33(6):29-36.

53. *'Popular antidepressants with good sleep effects include mirtazapine, amitriptyline, and agomelatine . . .'* Tobias Atkin, Stefano Comai and Gabriella Gobbi, (2018) 'Drugs for Insomnia beyond Benzodiazepines', *Pharmacological Reviews,* DOI: https://doi.org/10.1124/pr.117.014381

54. *'They have best evidence when there is insomnia and depression.'* Mi WF, Tabarak S, Wang L, Zhang SZ, Lin X, Du LT, Liu Z, Bao YP, Gao XJ, Zhang WH, Wang XQ, Fan TT, Li LZ, Hao XN, Fu Y, Shi Y, Guo LH, Sun HQ, Liu L, Si TM, Zhang HY, Lu L, Li SX (2020). 'Effects of agomelatine and mirtazapine on sleep disturbances in major depressive disorder: evidence from polysomnographic and resting-state functional connectivity analyses', *Sleep,* https://pubmed.ncbi.nlm.nih.gov/32406918/

55. *'They work by activating the GABA receptors in the brain, mimicking the GABA relaxation . . .'* Haefely W (1984). 'Benzodiazepine interactions with GABA receptors', *Neuroscience Letters.* https://pubmed.ncbi.nlm.nih.gov/6147796/

56. *'One 2020 study set out to look at the placebo effect . . .'* Yeung V, Sharpe L, Geers A, Colagiuri B (2020). 'Choice, Expectations, and the Placebo Effect for Sleep Difficulty'. *Annals of Behavioral Medicine.* https://pubmed.ncbi.nlm.nih.gov/31504091/

57. *'Epidemiological studies have linked eating more fish with better sleep.'* Liu J, Cui Y, Li L, Wu L, Hanlon A, Pinto-Martin J, Raine A, Hibbeln JR (2017). 'The mediating role of sleep in the fish consumption - cognitive functioning relationship: a cohort study'. *Scientific Reports,* https://www.nature.com/articles/s41598-017-17520-w

58. *'A randomised controlled trial in 2021 showed that 1 g of an omega-3 supplement twice daily . . .'* Behzad Nourosi, Erfan Naghsh, Sahar Esmaeil zadeh et al, (2021). 'Omega-3 in The Treatment of Mood and Sleep Disorders Induced by Hormone Therapy in Women with Breast Cancer: A Randomized, Double-Blinded, Placebo-Controlled Clinical Trial', PREPRINT (Version 1) available at Research Square [https://doi.org/10.21203/rs.3.rs-1055943/v1]

59. *'. . . but the jury is out on whether there's anything to worry about.'* Wehrein, P. (2013) 'High intake of omega-3 fats linked to increased prostate cancer risk.' *Harvard Health Publishing,* https://www.health.harvard.edu/blog/high-intake-of-omega-3-fats-linked-to-increased-prostate-cancer-risk-201308012009

60. *'In 2011 we got the results of a randomised, double-blind, placebo-controlled trial of 34 insomniacs.'* Zick SM, Wright BD, Sen A, Arnedt JT, (2011). 'Preliminary examination of the efficacy and safety of a standardized chamomile extract for chronic primary insomnia: a randomized placebo-controlled pilot study', *BMC Complementary Alternative Medicine.* https://www.ncbi.nlm.nih.gov/pmc/articles/PMC3198755/

61. *'A subsequent Australian study found that . . .'* Aspy DJ, Madden NA, Delfabbro P. (2108) 'Effects of Vitamin B6 (Pyridoxine) and a B Complex Preparation on Dreaming and Sleep'. *Perceptual and Motor Skills.* https://journals.sagepub.com/doi/10.1177/0031512518770326

62. *'Small studies have found that magnesium supplements may help people fall asleep quicker . . .'* Abbasi B, Kimiagar M, Sadeghniiat K, Shirazi MM, Hedayati M, Rashidkhani B. (2012) 'The effect of magnesium supplementation on primary insomnia in elderly: A double-blind placebo-controlled clinical trial'. *Journal of Research in Medical Science.* https://www.ncbi.nlm.nih.gov/pmc/articles/PMC3703169/

63. *'In tiny clinical trials Passiflora extracts showed anti-anxiety effects, including as a pre-med before surgery.'* Gregory WL, Mohr C, Pfankuch T, Soumyanath A. (2010) *'Passiflora incarnata L.* (Passionflower) extracts elicit GABA currents in hippocampal neurons in vitro, and show anxiogenic and anticonvulsant effects in vivo, varying with extraction method'. *Phytomedicine.* https://www.ncbi.nlm.nih.gov/pmc/articles/PMC2941540/
Movafegh A, Alizadeh R, Hajimohamadi F, Esfehani F, Nejatfar M. (2008) 'Preoperative oral Passiflora incarnata reduces anxiety in ambulatory surgery patients: a double-blind, placebo-controlled study'. *Anesthesia and Analgesia.* https://pubmed.ncbi.nlm.nih.gov/18499602/

64. *'And in mice it's a great sedative.'* Kim M, Lim HS, Lee HH, Kim TH (2017). 'Role Identification of Passiflora Incarnata Linnaeus: A Mini Review.' *Journal of Menopausal Medicine.* https://www.ncbi.nlm.nih.gov/pmc/articles/PMC5770524/

65. *'An Italian study gave a commercial preparation of lemon balm . . .'* Cases J, Ibarra A, Feuillère N, Roller M, Sukkar SG. (2011) 'Pilot trial of Melissa officinalis L. leaf extract in the treatment of volunteers suffering from mild-to-moderate anxiety disorders and sleep disturbances', *Mediterranean Journal of Nutrition and Metabolism,* https://www.ncbi.nlm.nih.gov/pmc/articles/PMC3230760/

66. *'In 2015, a meta-analysis of studies of valerian . . .'* Bent S, Padula A, Moore D, Patterson M, Mehling W. (2006) 'Valerian for sleep: a systematic review and meta-analysis'. *American Journal of Medicine.* https://www.ncbi.nlm.nih.gov/pmc/articles/PMC4394901/.

67. *'. . . a meta-analysis of 34 studies showed that aromatherapy . . .'* Cheong MJ, Kim S, Kim JS, Lee H, Lyu YS, Lee YR, Jeon B, Kang HW. (2021) 'A systematic literature review and meta-analysis of the clinical effects of aroma inhalation therapy on sleep problems', *Medicine (Baltimore),* https://www.ncbi.nlm.nih.gov/pmc/articles/PMC7939222/

68. *'In a randomised, controlled trial of 50 residents . . .'* Chawla J, (2022) 'Acupressure for Insomnia', Medscape, https://emedicine.medscape.com/article/1187829-treatment#d11

69. *'Cannabis plants and derivatives that have less than 0.3 per cent THC are classified as 'hemp'.* Shannon S, Lewis N, Lee H, Hughes S. (2019)'Cannabidiol in Anxiety and Sleep: A Large Case Series'. *The Permanente Journal,* https://www.ncbi.nlm.nih.gov/pmc/articles/PMC6326553/

70. *'In a 2020 study of older adults with chronic pain . . .'* Sznitman SR, Vulfsons S, Meiri D, Weinstein G. (2020) 'Medical cannabis and insomnia in older adults with chronic pain: a cross-sectional study', *BMJ Support Palliative Care,* https://pubmed.ncbi.nlm.nih.gov/31959585/

71. *'Separately, a 2020 meta-analysis of five studies . . .'* Bhagavan C, Kung S, Doppen M, John M, Vakalalabure I, Oldfield K, Braithwaite I, Newton-Howes G. (2020) 'Cannabinoids in the Treatment of Insomnia Disorder: A Systematic Review and Meta-Analysis.' *CNS Drugs,* https://pubmed.ncbi.nlm.nih.gov/33244728/

72. *'A 2022 paper suggested that because . . .'* Kolla BP, Hayes L, Cox C, Eatwell L, Deyo-Svendsen M, Mansukhani MP. (2022) 'The Effects of Cannabinoids on Sleep', *Journal of Primary Care and Community Health,* https://www.ncbi.nlm.nih.gov/pmc/articles/PMC9036386/

73. *'. . . we know from studies that non-painkiller options work.'* Harvard Health Publishing (2017) https://www.health.harvard.edu/pain/8-non-invasive-pain-relief-techniques-that-really-work

74. *'Studies show musculoskeletal symptoms can hit up to 80 per cent of women going through menopause.'* Yang YL, Chee W, Im EO. (2019) 'Type 2 Diabetes and Musculoskeletal Symptoms Among Midlife Women'. *Diabetes Education.* https://www.ncbi.nlm.nih.gov/pmc/articles/PMC6750959/

75. *'. . . but there is some evidence that hormone replacement therapy can help.'* Caleigh Tate, Showchuk,

Endnotes

University of Regina, Saskatchewan (2020) 'The Effect of Postmenopausal Hormone Therapy on the Prevalence of Musculoskeletal Pain Conditions: A Systematic Review and Meta-Analysis' https://ourspace.uregina.ca/bitstream/handle/10294/11852/Showchuk_2021_PsychThesis.pdf?sequence=1

76. *'It stuffs up the quality of your sleep.'* He S, Hasler BP, Chakravorty S (2019). 'Alcohol and sleep-related problems', *Current Opinion Psychology.* https://www.ncbi.nlm.nih.gov/pmc/articles/PMC6801009/

77. *'Scientists break down napping into three types.'* Lastella M, Halson SL, Vitale JA, Memon AR, Vincent GE. (2021) 'To Nap or Not to Nap? A Systematic Review Evaluating Napping Behavior in Athletes and the Impact on Various Measures of Athletic Performance', *Natural Science Sleep.* https://www.ncbi.nlm.nih.gov/pmc/articles/PMC8238550/

78. *'Long nappers are also more likely to be obese . . .'* Leng Y, Redline S, Stone KL, Ancoli-Israel S, Yaffe K. (2019) 'Objective napping, cognitive decline, and risk of cognitive impairment in older men'. *Alzheimer's and Dementia.* https://www.ncbi.nlm.nih.gov/pmc/articles/PMC6699896/

79. *'One Japanese study found that napping for less than 30 minutes . . .'* Kitamura, K., Watanabe, Y., Nakamura, K. et al (2021). 'Short daytime napping reduces the risk of cognitive decline in community-dwelling older adults: a 5-year longitudinal study'. *BMC Geriatrics* Vol 21, https://bmcgeriatr.biomedcentral.com/articles/10.1186/s12877-021-02418-0#citeas

80. *'Another 2011 study found that taking a nap . . .'* Gujar N, McDonald SA, Nishida M, Walker MP, (2011), 'A role for REM sleep in recalibrating the sensitivity of the human brain to specific emotions', *Cerebral Cortex*, https://www.ncbi.nlm.nih.gov/pmc/articles/PMC3000566/

81. *'Some studies have found that napping beyond an hour . . .'* Monk TH, Buysse DJ, Carrier J, Billy BD, Rose LR (2001). 'Effects of afternoon "siesta" naps on sleep, alertness, performance, and circadian rhythms in the elderly', *Sleep*, https://pubmed.ncbi.nlm.nih.gov/11560181/

Chapter 10

1. *'Women are 55 per cent more likely to get dementia than men . . .'* Gilsanz P, Lee C, Corrada MM, Kawas CH, Quesenberry CP Jr, Whitmer RA. (2019) 'Reproductive period and risk of dementia in a diverse cohort of health care members.' *Neurology*, https://www.ncbi.nlm.nih.gov/pmc/articles/PMC6511081/

2. *'Some studies have found that men and women have the same rate of dementia up to age 80 . . .'* Beam CR, Kaneshiro C, Jang JY, Reynolds CA, Pedersen NL, Gatz M. (2018) 'Differences Between Women and Men in Incidence Rates of Dementia and Alzheimer's Disease.' *Journal of Alzheimer's Disease*, https://www.ncbi.nlm.nih.gov/pmc/articles/PMC6226313/

3. *'A recent study found that around the world, women's reduced access to education . . .'* Bloomberg M, Dugravot A, Dumurgier J, Kivimaki M, Fayosse A, Steptoe A, Britton A, Singh-Manoux A, Sabia S. (2021) 'Sex differences and the role of education in cognitive ageing: analysis of two UK-based prospective cohort studies', *Lancet Public Health*, https://www.ncbi.nlm.nih.gov/pmc/articles/PMC8141610/

4. *'One 2019 study in the journal* Neurology *reported on almost 16,000 women . . .'* Gilsanz P, Lee C, Corrada MM, Kawas CH, Quesenberry CP Jr, Whitmer RA (2019). 'Reproductive period and risk of dementia in a diverse cohort of health care members', *Neurology*, https://www.ncbi.nlm.nih.gov/pmc/articles/PMC6511081/

5. *'Animal studies indicate that oestrogen influences the organisation . . '* Bailey ME, Wang AC, Hao J, Janssen WG, Hara Y, Dumitriu D, Hof PR, Morrison JH, (2011). 'Interactive effects of age and estrogen on cortical neurons: implications for cognitive aging', *Neuroscience.* https://www.ncbi.nlm.nih.gov/pmc/articles/PMC3166405/

6. *'It also seems to be an actual neurotransmitter.'* 'Brian P. Kenealy, Amita Kapoor, Kathryn A. Guerriero, Kim L. Keen, James P. Garcia, Joseph R. Kurian, Toni E. Ziegler, Ei Terasawa, (2013) 'Neuroestradiol in the Hypothalamus Contributes to the Regulation of Gonadotropin Releasing Hormone Release', *Journal of Neuroscience*, https://www.jneurosci.org/content/33/49/19051

7. *'Specifically, the most significant effect of oestrogen on cognitive function . . .'* Cutter WJ, Norbury R, Murphy DGM (2003), 'Oestrogen, brain function, and neuropsychiatric disorders', *Journal of Neurology, Neurosurgery & Psychiatry*, https://jnnp.bmj.com/content/74/7/837

8. *'. . . which is a broad term for memories that come from what you read or hear.'* Tatsumi, I.F., Watanabe, M. (2009). 'Verbal Memory'. In: Binder, M.D., Hirokawa, N., Windhorst, U. (eds) *Encyclopedia of Neuroscience*. Springer, Berlin, Heidelberg. https://doi.org/10.1007/978-3-540-29678-2_6266

9. *'Progesterone has a significant protective effect in the brain . . .'* Guennoun R. (2020) 'Progesterone in the Brain: Hormone, Neurosteroid and Neuroprotectant', *International Journal of Molecular Science*, https://www.ncbi.nlm.nih.gov/pmc/articles/PMC7432434/

10. *'This phase lasts between 4.37 and 8.57 years and it's the phase I call hormone hell.'* Paramsothy P, Harlow SD, Nan B, Greendale GA, Santoro N, Crawford SL, Gold EB, Tepper PG, Randolph JF Jr. (2017) 'Duration of the menopausal transition is longer in women with young age at onset: the multiethnic Study of Women's Health Across the Nation.' *Menopause*, https://journals.lww.com/menopausejournal/Abstract/2017/02000/Duration_of_the_menopausal_transition_is_longer_in.5.aspx

11. *'During this time your hormone levels are literally all over the show and blood tests are uninterpretable . . .'* Santoro N, Randolph JF Jr. (2011) 'Reproductive hormones and the menopause transition', *Obstetrics and Gynecology Clinics of North America*, https://www.ncbi.nlm.nih.gov/pmc/articles/PMC3197715/

12. *'Unlike the yo-yoing oestrogen levels, progesterone levels also decline but do so gradually during perimenopause.'* Davis, S., Lambrinoudaki, I., Lumsden, M. et al, (2015), 'Menopause', *Nature Reviews Disease Primers*, https://doi.org/10.1038/nrdp.2015.4

13. *'. . . as a rule, brain fog is a perimenopause problem . . .'* Jett S, Malviya N, Schelbaum E, Jang G, Jahan E, Clancy K, Hristov H, Pahlajani S, Niotis K, Loeb-Zeitlin S, Havryliuk Y, Isaacson R, Brinton RD and Mosconi L (2022) 'Endogenous and Exogenous Estrogen Exposures: How Women's Reproductive Health Can Drive Brain Aging and Inform Alzheimer's Prevention'. *Frontiers in Aging Neuroscience*, https://www.frontiersin.org/articles/10.3389/fnagi.2022.831807/full#h3

14. *'In a huge US study published in 2013 . . .'* Epperson CN, Sammel MD, Freeman EW (2013). 'Menopause effects on verbal memory: findings from a longitudinal community cohort.' *Journal of Clinical Endocrinology and Metabolism*, https://www.ncbi.nlm.nih.gov/pmc/articles/PMC3763981/

15. *'That's because studies have found the worse your hot flushes . . .'* Drogos LL, Rubin LH, Geller SE, Banuvar S, Shulman LP, Maki PM (2013). 'Objective cognitive performance is related to subjective memory complaints in midlife women with moderate to severe vasomotor symptoms', *Menopause*, https://www.ncbi.nlm.nih.gov/pmc/articles/PMC3762921/

16. *'Perimenopause is the highest risk time for women to experience a mood disorder.'* Bromberger JT, Kravitz HM, Chang YF, Cyranowski JM, Brown C, Matthews KA (2011). 'Major depression during and after the menopausal transition: Study of Women's Health Across the Nation (SWAN)', *Psychological Medicine*, https://www.ncbi.nlm.nih.gov/pmc/articles/PMC3584692/

17. *'However, small trials say yes.'* Maki P, Berga S. (2021), https://imswebinars.com/brain-function-in-the-menopause-where-do-we-stand-now

18. *'But the Women's Health Initiative also found that women aged 65 years . . .'* Maki P, Manson, J (2021) 'Menopausal hormone therapy and dementia'. *The BMJ Opinion*, https://blogs.bmj.com/bmj/2021/09/29/menopausal-hormone-therapy-and-dementia/

19. *'Studies show that women who start HRT early have better memory.'* Australian menopause Society, https://www.menopause.org.au/hp/information-sheets/oestrogen-and-cognition-in-the-perimenopause-and-menopause

20. *'In 2021, a meta-analysis of 24 trials found that the majority of studies found that taking HRT . . .'* Petra Stute, Johanna Wienges, Anne-Sophie Koller, Christina Giese, Wiebke Wesemüller, Heidrun Janka, Sabrina Baumgartner, (2021) 'Cognitive health after menopause: Does menopausal hormone therapy affect it?', *Best Practice & Research Clinical Endocrinology & Metabolism*, https://doi.org/10.1016/j.beem.2021.101565.

Endnotes

21. *'If that's you, you should absolutely be on HRT until age 51 . . .'* Magraith K, Stuckey B, (2019) 'Making choices at Menopause', *Australian Journal of General Practice*, doi: 10.31128/AJGP-02-19-4851

22. *'Testosterone, the main male hormone, is made by Leydig cells . . .'* Cai Z and Li H (2020) 'An Updated Review: Androgens and Cognitive Impairment in Older Men'. *Frontiers in Endocrinology*, https://www.frontiersin.org/articles/10.3389/fendo.2020.586909/full

23. *'After the age of 40 years, men have a 1.6 per cent decline in testosterone levels each year.'* Hua JT, Hildreth KL, Pelak VS. (2016) 'Effects of Testosterone Therapy on Cognitive Function in Aging: A Systematic Review'. *Cognitive and Behavioral Neurology*. https://www.ncbi.nlm.nih.gov/pmc/articles/PMC5079177/

24. *'Studies in men . . .'* Beauchet O. (2006) 'Testosterone and cognitive function: current clinical evidence of a relationship'. *European Society of Endocrinology EJE*. https://eje.bioscientifica.com/view/journals/eje/155/6/1550773.xml

25. *'. . . lots of super common chronic diseases can cause low testosterone levels.'* Irene Chan, Mark Ng, Tang Fui, Jeffrey D Zajac, Mathis Grossmann, (2014) 'Assessment and management of male androgen disorders: an update' *Australian Family Physician*, https://www.racgp.org.au/afp/2014/may/male-androgen-disorders

26. *'. . . where getting the diagnosis of testosterone deficiency is sooo difficult, that lots of doctors give up.'* Irene Chan, Mark Ng, Tang Fui, Jeffrey D Zajac, Mathis Grossmann, (2014) 'Assessment and management of male androgen disorders: an update' *Australian Family Physician*, https://www.racgp.org.au/afp/2014/may/male-androgen-disorders

27. *'Certainly there are trials that show that . . .'* Cai Z and Li H (2020) 'An Updated Review: Androgens and Cognitive Impairment in Older Men'. *Frontiers in Endocrinology*, https://www.frontiersin.org/articles/10.3389/fendo.2020.586909/full

28. *'But a 2019 meta-analysis of 23 trials found pretty . . .'* Cecilie R Buskbjerg, Claus H Gravholt, Helene R Dalby, Ali Amidi, Robert Zachariae, (2019) 'Testosterone Supplementation and Cognitive Functioning in Men—A Systematic Review and Meta-Analysis', *Journal of the Endocrine Society*, https://doi.org/10.1210/js.2019-00119

29. *'These include increased risk of blood clots, prostate problems, breast enlargement, mood swings and aggression, decreased testicle size and worsening of sleep apnoea.'* Grech A, Breck J, Heidelbaugh J. (2014) 'Adverse effects of testosterone replacement therapy: an update on the evidence and controversy', *Therapeutic Advances in Drug Safety*, https://www.ncbi.nlm.nih.gov/pmc/articles/PMC4212439/

Index

Note: page numbers in *italics* refer to illustrations.

Index

Index

Index